Fogel MDavis

State College

December 1981

Commissurotomy
Consciousness
and Unity of Mind

Charles E. Marks

A Bradford Book

The MIT Press
Cambridge, Massachusetts
London, England

Second printing, 1981

Printed in the United States of America

Library of Congress catalog card number 81-84119
ISBN 0-262-63076-1 (paper)

Contents

The Split-Brain Syndrome: An Example of the Philosophically Puzzling Behavior Resulting from
Commissurotomy   3

How to Generate Philosophical Problems about
Split-Brains   6

Preliminary Analysis and Some Strategy   10

In What Sense Do Split-Brain Patients Lack Unity
of Consciousness?   12

Is the Consciousness of Split-Brain Patients Always
Disunified?   17

Can a Single Mind Ever Have a Disunified Consciousness?   30

Some Rough Truth Conditions for 'Split-Brain
Patients Have One (Two) Mind(s)'   33

How Does Disunity of Consciousness Bear upon
Unity of Mind?   35

Will an Adequate Psychology Favor a One-Mind
Account of Split-Brain Patients?   40

Wittgensteinian Postscript   43

Notes   46

Bibliography   52

Commissurotomy, Consciousness and Unity of Mind

"I thus drew steadily nearer to that truth, by whose partial discovery I have been doomed to such dreadful shipwreck: that man is not truly one, but truly two. I say two, because the state of my knowledge does not pass beyond that point. Others will follow, others will outstrip me on the same lines; and I hazard the guess that man will ultimately be known for a mere polity of multifarious, incongruous and independent denizens." *Dr. Jekyll and Mr. Hyde*

" 'Ah, I begin to see the light,' broke in McNeil. 'If communication occurs on such a scale then it becomes somewhat doubtful whether we should talk anymore of separate individuals!' " *The Black Cloud*

"When we do philosophy we are like savages, primitive people, who hear the expressions of civilized men, put a false interpretation on them, and then draw the queerest conclusions from it." *Philosophical Investigations*

Recent psychological studies of commissurotomy patients[1] have provoked considerable, sometimes wild, speculation by both philosophers and the experimenters themselves. Among neuropsychologists,[2] the prevalent view is that the split-brain patient has two minds. These two minds are taken to exemplify a variety of dichotomies: for example, one is atomistic, analytic, digital, symbolic, discursive; the other, holistic, synthetic, analogic, perceptual, eidetic. Further, it is inferred, there is a similar split in the fundamental cognitive styles of the left and right halves of the intact brain,[3] whether or not they are also counted as separate minds. Philosophers have been no less extravagant. The split-brain studies reveal, Puccetti[4] claims, that we, like split-brain patients, are collectives of two minds and persons, although we tend to identify with the more articulate member. Nagel[5] thinks that the research shows that our concept of the unity of a person is in disarray and that this concept, along with other mentalistic concepts, may be incompatible with an understanding of the physical basis of mind.

In this monograph, my primary concern is the number of minds split-brain patients have; the speculations on what types of minds these may be, deriving from experiments on lateral specialization and cerebral dominance, are left for another time. I advocate a conservative assessment of split-brain research: the split-brain patient has one mind and is one person, although he has on occasion a disunified consciousness. The experimental results pose no special threat to our concept of the unity of a person; but they do falsify the common belief that a single mind can always jointly introspect its simultaneous conscious contents.

The striking philosophical claims they have occasioned, as well as their intrinsic interest, obviously recommend the split-brain studies to philosophers. But there is another reason for philosophers to reflect on the split-brain research that may be concealed in works which, like the present one, do not contain much experimental or neurological detail. In order to characterize the results of split-brain research, one must make a great number of difficult, detailed decisions on the relation of specific, usually messy, behavioral and neurological data to mentalistic description. Rather than helping, the traditional theories of mind seem hopelessly out of place. The mind-body problem looks surprisingly different in close-up; the change of perspective is both disconcerting and stimulating.

THE SPLIT-BRAIN SYNDROME: AN EXAMPLE
OF THE PHILOSOPHICALLY PUZZLING BEHAVIOR
RESULTING FROM COMMISSUROTOMY

Although there were earlier studies and research is conducted else-
where, the most extensive psychological studies of split-brain patients have been done by Roger Sperry and his coworkers at the
California Institute of Technology. The subjects involved in this
research are patients of J. E. Bogen, of the Ross-Loos Medical
Group, and P. J. Vogel, Chief of Neurosurgery at the White Me-
morial Medical Center in Los Angeles. As of 1974, sixteen commissurotomies had been performed in a series which began in the
early 1960s; but the sample involved in the psychological studies is
closer to six, chosen in part because they had minimal brain damage other than that directly linked to the operation.

The operation, which consists of the sectioning of the corpus
callosum and other minor commissures linking the two cerebral
hemispheres,[6] is undertaken for the relief of uncontrollable epilepsy. Medically, it is considered a success. Epileptic attacks became less frequent, were confined to one hemisphere, or
disappeared entirely. In fact, Sperry assures us that "a person two
years recovered from the operation and otherwise without compli-
cations might easily go through a routine medical checkup without
revealing that anything was wrong to someone not acquainted
with his surgical history."[7]

The psychological result is less clear. After recovery from the
operation, the patients' behavior is, by and large, normal. If you
knew them before the operation, you would not notice any dra-
matic changes in their intellect, personality, or day-to-day behavior.
It is not just that such observation is likely to be too casual to de-
tect a difference. In a number of clinical papers published in the

1940s, Akelaitis [8] recorded his failure to find any interesting psychological result attributable to a series of partial and total commissurotomies. This surprising lack of effect prompted McCulloch's pessimistic remark that the sole function of the corpus callosum was to transmit epileptic seizures from one hemisphere to the other. [9] Yet, under controlled conditions, the behavior of split-brain patients is decidedly abnormal. When input is limited to, and response demand placed on, one of the hemispheres, it has seemed to various experimenters that they were dealing with "two separate spheres of conscious awareness, two separate conscious entities or minds running in parallel in the same cranium, each with its own sensations, perceptions, cognitive processes, learning experiences, memories, and so on." [10]

The abnormal behavior of split-brain patients in such controlled conditions is illustrated by the following. A subject, S, is told to fixate a point on a screen before him. 'Key ring' is flashed on the screen for a tenth of a second, with 'key' appearing to the left of the fixation point and 'ring' to the right. Since the time is too brief for eye movement, information from the right visual field ('ring') is projected exclusively to the left hemisphere and information from the left visual field ('key') is projected exclusively to the right hemisphere. [11] If S is asked to say what he saw, he responds that he saw 'ring.' Questioned about what kind of ring, he is as likely to say that it is a wedding ring, a boxing ring, the ring of a bell, as that it is a key ring. S's verbal responses show no awareness of 'key.' On the other hand, if S is instead asked to retrieve, with his left hand, what he saw from an array of items (concealed from sight), he will retrieve a key while rejecting all varieties of rings. Similarly, if S is asked to point with his left hand to what he saw, he will point to a key (or a picture of a key) and not to a ring (or a picture of a ring). S's response with his left hand indicates an awareness of 'key,' but none of 'ring.' If S is asked to sort through an array of items (concealed from sight) with both hands and pick out what he saw, the right and left hands work independently. The right hand will pick up and reject a key before settling on a ring; the left will pick up and reject a ring before settling on a key. In general, when the response demanded is controlled by the left hemisphere, it indicates that S was aware of 'ring' and unaware of 'key'; when the response demanded is controlled by the right hemisphere, it indicates that S was aware of 'key' and unaware of 'ring.' Someone seems to have seen 'key' and someone seems to have seen 'ring' and they seem unaware of each other. No one is aware of seeing 'key ring.'

One other feature of our example is worth remarking on. Even the simple tasks demanded of the minor[12] hemisphere implicate a wide range of psychological functions. The instructions to pick out what is named must be perceived and understood, 'key' must be perceived and understood to name keys, the key must be identified by touch, and so on. According to Sperry,[13] the performance of such a task is beyond the capacity of a chimp; the range and integration of functions demanded is characteristically human.

The standard explanation of the sort of behavior exhibited is roughly as follows: The left half of the field of vision is conveyed to the right side of the brain, and vice versa. Thus the right brain sees only the word 'key' and the left brain sees only the word 'ring.' The right brain is mute, and so the oral response to the question, by the left brain, reports only what the left brain saw, the word 'ring.' The left hand is controlled by the right brain; so it points to what is named by the word the right brain saw, a key. In discussion of such experiments, the right and left brain are commonly said, with varying degrees of caution, to see, reach, remember, and the like. They are thus treated as subjects of experience, i.e., as separate persons. And the explanation for the failure to elicit any response suggesting that 'key ring' has been or is known to have occurred is that the subjects of the two experiences, the seeing of 'key' and the seeing of 'ring,' are not the same and not, because of sectioning of the corpus callosum and the experimental controls, in communication with each other. [14]

With suitable controls, it is also possible to confine input from the other senses, except taste, to a single hemisphere. The abnormalities in the behavior of split-brain patients that arise when input is limited to, and response demand placed on, one hemisphere have now been extensively mapped. These abnormalities constitute the bulk of "the syndrome of the neocortical commissures" or, as I shall call it, the split-brain syndrome.[15] The extent of the abnormalities exhibited varies with the type of surgery the patient undergoes, with whether the corpus callosum and all the minor commissures are totally severed.[16] Even when the corpus callosum and the minor commissures have been completely sectioned, as for all of Vogel and Bogen's patients, there are sizable individual differences among patients; and there are equally sizable differences between the immediate postoperative behavior of individual patients and their later behavior.[17] One patient, for example, was able to read across midline seven years after the operation, although he was unable to do this postoperatively. So, seven years after the operation, this patient would not even exhibit the kind of behavior illustrated in the "key ring" example. Fortunately, the fine grain of empirical fact, as well as its markedly individual character, is largely irrelevant to my philosophical purposes. Accordingly, I will treat all split-brain patients as though they had a complete commissurotomy and exhibited the complete syndrome. The "key ring" experiments will be used throughout to illustrate the kind of behavior that leads to philosophical difficulties.

HOW TO GENERATE PHILOSOPHICAL
PROBLEMS ABOUT SPLIT-BRAINS

Behavior of the sort illustrated by the "key ring" experiment is the starting point for a chain of inferences which generates the philosophical problems that are my main concern. The most important steps along the way are:

(1) S exhibits the split-brain syndrome.

(2) S has two independent streams of consciousness (or a disunified consciousness).

(3) S has two minds.

(4) S is two persons (or contains two subjects of experience).

(5) Human beings with commissures intact have two minds, are
two persons (contain two subjects of experience) as well.

In outline, the argument linking these propositions together runs
as follows.

Consider the behavior directed by the right hemisphere of a
split-brain patient in the "key ring" experiment. He points, with
his left hand to a picture of a key when asked to point to what he
saw, retrieves with his left hand a key from an array of items when
asked to retrieve what he saw, and so on. If a person with commissures intact exhibited similar behavior, there would be no doubt
that conscious mental activity was involved. There is no reason to
doubt that this is true in the split-brain case as well, at least no
reason which does not generalize to a reason for skepticism about
other minds or the consciousness of mutes. So there are conscious
mental processes associated with minor-hemisphere activity in
split-brain patients.

Do these events belong to a single stream of consciousness? Intuitively, two simultaneous conscious mental events belong to the
same stream of consciousness only if some introspective awareness
encompasses both of them. In the "key ring" experiment, someone is directly aware of seeing 'key'; and at the same time, someone is directly aware of seeing 'ring.' But no one is directly aware
that both are seen, that these two mental events occurred simultaneously. So, at least in this experimental setup, there are two
independent streams of consciousness. The cause of this disunity
in consciousness is the commissurotomy the patients underwent.
Since the commissures remain severed, whether in the laboratory
or at home, these patients always have two independent streams
of consciousness. The fact that, outside the laboratory, their

behavior does not indicate two streams of consciousness is explained by the large overlap in the contents of the two streams. In the case of vision, for example, normal eye movement would largely suffice to duplicate visual experience in each hemisphere. If, in the "key ring" experiment, 'key ring' were projected long enough to allow eye movement, about 250 milliseconds, then both hemispheres would see 'key' and 'ring' and there would be no behavior indicative of a split in consciousness. Yet, as the "key ring" experiment shows, there would still be two seeings of 'key' and 'ring.' Since the normal environment of split-brain patients does not present objects for just a tenth of a second, there is plenty of time for eye movement, thus ensuring a duplication of visual experience and the lack of any behavior that would indicate a disunity in consciousness. In addition to eye movement, several other factors contribute to the overlap of the contents of each stream of consciousness and so explain the normalcy of the split-brain patient's everyday behavior.

The arguments from (2) to (3) and from (3) to (4) are relatively simple. Each hemisphere, as far as psychological function goes, is pretty much full service. To be sure, there are significant differences: for example, the right hemisphere cannot produce speech, though it can comprehend it, and the left is not very good at a variety of spatial tasks. But both can learn, remember, express emotion, and so on, at a characteristically human level. The activity each supports seems broad enough, complex enough, and organized enough to characterize a human mind.[18] The reason for saying that these patients have two minds is that neither hemisphere (or its associated mind) has access to the contents of the other in the way it has access to its own contents. Each has its own experiences which it knows directly; it learns of the experiences of the other in ways not different in principle from the ways we learn about our friends.[19] If a person is taken to be an embodied mind with a certain degree of complexity and organization, then split-brain patients are two persons, since they embody two minds of the requisite sort.

Before the operation, the cerebral commissures of the split-brain patients were intact just as ours are. If the best explanation of why the split-brain patient has two minds after the operation requires that he had two preoperatively, then we have two minds as well.[20] The argument, thus far, is that split-brain patients have two minds, contain two subjects of experience after commissurotomy. Call these LB and RB (where LB is the one associated with the left hemisphere, RB the one associated with the right). If there were not two minds before the operation, then either one of these is the new mind or they both are.

If one of RB and LB is the new mind, which is it? Presumably, RB is the new mind and LB persists through the operation. Although LB's capacities have diminished somewhat, he can articulate, and so seems to remember, the patient's previous actions, experiences, and so on. The trouble is that RB also seems to remember the patient's previous actions and experiences—at least if he is given suitable tests (e.g., asked to point to a picture of where he went to school).[21] It seems that there is no principled way of choosing which of them persists through the operation: if one of them is the old mind, so is the other. In addition, if a choice is made, say the RB is the new mind, it seems impossible to explain the postoperative capacities and apparent memories of the alleged new mind without implicating its existence before the operation. For example, when did RB learn how to understand English, what a key was, and so forth? That disposes of the possibility that just one of RB and LB is the new mind.

The second alternative is that neither RB nor LB existed before the operation. The main problem with this alternative is how to explain why neither existed although the physiological basis for both did. Suppose that, before the operation, the sole subject of experience was EB (who is identical with neither LB nor RB). Consider what happens if the "key ring" experiment is performed *before* the commissurotomy. If EB is the sole subject of experience, then there is no 'key'-seeing which is not a part of 'key ring'-seeing. But this is puzzling. The right and left hemispheres have been stimulated in just the way that, in the absence of the commissures, is sufficient to produce a 'key'-seeing experience in RB and a 'ring'-seeing experience in LB. The usual explanation is that, with the callosum intact, the right hemisphere is made aware that the left is seeing 'ring' and perhaps even brought to have such an experience (and vice versa).[22] But then it looks as though the difference between the normal and split-brain cases is mainly one of *communication*. In the normal human being, the two hemispheres communicate directly through the corpus callosum; in the split-brain base, they must rely at best on peripheral and subcortical mechanisms. But then why do we not have two subjects of experience, RB and LB, *before* the commissurotomy who communicate through the corpus callosum?

So it looks as though, if there are two subjects of experience after the commissurotomy, there were two before as well. Since we are in the same state as the split-brain patients before the operation, we contain two subjects of experience as well.

That completes my sketch of the arguments that are supposed to take us from (1) to (5), from the indisputable behavior of split-brain patients under controlled conditions to the nearly incredible claim that we are all two. The extended argument is an amalgam and reconstruction of various arguments, explicit and implicit in the literature; and not everyone who starts down the path goes all the way. Eccles, for example, thinks that (2) does not follow from (1) because minor hemisphere processes are not conscious.[23] MacKay does not get to (3) because, he believes, there is a single control center for the separate streams of consciousness.[24] Bogen,[25] using the queer formula "two minds in one person," stops short of (4) in letter if not in spirit. Perhaps only a philosopher, Puccetti, for example, can take the whole trip self-consciously.

PRELIMINARY ANALYSIS AND SOME STRATEGY

The problem is whether the chain of inferences sketched above stops at a philosophically comfortable point. It is obvious that the completed chain poses a philosophical problem. If nothing else, we do believe that each of us is a single agent acting upon the world, a single locus of responsibility, a single subject of experience, and not a collective. It is also fairly plain that, even if one can stop at the point of thinking that split-brain subjects, but not us, are two, there are problems as well. Imagine that the notorious Martian supersurgeons performed undetected commissurotomies on all of us last year as part of a sinister (but misguided) plot to produce a population explosion. Thanks to their fabled technology, recovery was nearly instantaneous; there was no additional brain damage, and so on. If the split-brain patients are a rough guide, our behavior—including our introspective reports—would have been pretty much as it actually was. Of course, if we become subjects for Sperry's experiments, we would behave like split-brain patients; and if the proper x-rays were taken, the operation would be disclosed. For my part, I find it scarcely conceivable that my individuality depends upon the falsity of this surgical fantasy or upon any facts about how I might behave in the "key ring" experiment. On the other hand, the actual laboratory results with split-brain subjects have to be confronted. In the "key ring" experiments, someone seems to see 'key' and someone seems to see 'ring,' and they appear to be strangers. So there are philosophical difficulties even if the inference from 'Split-brain patients are two' to 'We're all two, too' fails.

Starting at the beginning of the chain, it is implausible that the mental processes associated with the minor hemisphere in these patients are all unconscious, nor as I shall later show, would this help.[26] And it does seem correct that the behavior of split-brain patients, under experimental conditions, shows that their consciousness is disunified in some sense. The crux is whether the sense in which, and the extent to which, split-brain patients lack unity of consciousness implies that they have two minds.

This suggests the following strategy. First, specify the sense in which the consciousness of split-brain patients is disunified. If, contrary to what is usually thought, there is no compelling reason to think that disunity is a standing condition, the case for two minds is considerably weakened, even if one accepts a basically Cartesian picture of mind. At least, it is considerably weakened if Nagel is wrong in thinking that the ordinary, unanalyzed concept of mind cannot tolerate even occasional disunity.[27] So Nagel's claim must be assessed. That is about as far as one can go when relying on an intuitive understanding of what minds are. If all goes well, the result will be that split-brain patients do not always have a disunified consciousness and a single mind can, on occasion, have a disunified consciousness. But the main question still remains: can a single mind tolerate a consciousness disunified to the extent of split-brain patients? At this point, one needs a theory of mind. At least, one needs enough of an account, however rough, to suggest and motivate something like the relevant truth conditions for 'Split-brain patients have one (two) mind(s).' These in hand, one hopes that the relation of facts about disunity in consciousness to unity of mind will be clear enough to provide the basis for a principled decision on the split-brain patients. This is the strategy I pursue, with varying degrees of detail and perseverance, in what follows.

IN WHAT SENSE DO SPLIT-BRAIN PATIENTS LACK UNITY OF CONSCIOUSNESS?

Split-brain patients differ from us anatomically; and in a variety of test conditions, they differ from us behaviorally as well. The differences in behavior are supposed to show that their conscious states are related in ways unlike ours: they are said to lack unity of consciousness, have a disunified consciousness, have separate spheres of consciousness, or have two independent streams of consciousness. As a partial explication of what might be meant,

I shall offer a rough necessary condition for two simultaneous conscious experiences belonging to the same unified consciousness. If it is to be useful, it must satisfy the following conditions: (1) It should be a plausible necessary condition for a person having a unified consciousness at a given time on *some* intuitive understanding of 'unified consciousness.' (2) The behavior exhibited by split-brain patients should be clearly relevant to showing that the condition is failed. (3) It should be plausible that the condition is never, or almost never failed by people whose commissures are intact. At a minimum, their behavior in experiments like the "key ring" experiment should not be evidence that the condition is failed. (4) Finally, it should be possible to determine whether split-brain patients fail the condition without first deciding how many minds they have or how many subjects of experience they contain.

Consider, again, the "key ring" experiment. Unless we prejudge the issue of how many subjects the split-brain patient contains, his behavior, like that of a normal control, indicates that he is aware of seeing 'key' and that he is aware of seeing 'ring.' The difference is that his behavior indicates that he, unlike a normal control, is not aware of seeing *both* 'key' and 'ring.' This suggests a rough necessary condition for two simultaneous conscious experiences belonging to the same stream of consciousness: e_1 and e_2 belong to the same unified consciousness only if they are known, by introspection, to be simultaneous. 'Introspection' is here used descriptively, to refer to that kind of apparently noninferential knowledge a person has of his own conscious mental states. One clear sense, then, in which the split-brain subject in the "key ring" experiment lacks a unified consciousness is that no one is introspectively aware that the 'key'-seeing experience and the 'ring'-seeing experience are simultaneous.[28]

I think that the proposed condition captures the fundamental sense in which split-brain patients do, at least some of the time, lack unity of consciousness. The other facts which are occasionally used to illustrate the split-brain subject's disunified conscious-ness—e.g., the lack of a unified visual field, the failure to integrate visual experiences, the failure to experience the simpler relations between simultaneous mental events—are obvious consequences of the subject's stream of consciousness being split in the way the condition describes. There is, of course, behavioral evidence for other separations in the mental lives of split-brain patients which, though not themselves divisions in consciousness, may give rise to disunity in consciousness. For example, the "key ring" experiment forces us to suppose that short-term memory[29] is sometimes lateralized, at least in part. The actual divisions in consciousness consequent upon other mental separations will be captured by the proposed condition.

I considered, and with some misgivings rejected, a weaker neces-sary condition for unity of consciousness (borrowed from Grice):[30] two simultaneous conscious experiences, e_1 and e_2, belong to the same unified consciousness only if they would, given certain con-ditions, be known, by memory or introspection, to be simultan-eous. The following sort of possible case (due to John Perry) argues for the inclusion of memory: I am grading papers and lis-tening to some music on the radio. I am aware of the paper I am grading. If you asked, I could tell you about, for example, the cur-ious substitution of 'Touring machine' for 'Turing machine.' I am also aware of the music. If you asked, I could tell you about the funny quality of the singer's voice. But I am not, as far as my introspection goes, aware that I am aware of both. We believe that, if I had tried, I could have had such awareness. But is this true? No doubt I could have been aware that I was simultaneously aware of *some* features of the music and the paper. But is it obvious that this was possible for the very *same* features I in fact attended to? Our capacity for simultaneous attention may set limits to our abilities to monitor such attention. If we are so limited, it appears that, on my account, we may all have on occasion a disunified consciousness; and this seems an unduly paradoxical response to a possible, humdrum empirical fact. On the other hand, I do know, by memory, that I was attending both to the misprint and the funny quality of the singer's voice. So the inclusion of memory seems reasonable.

A similar kind of case favors weakening the requirement to 'would be known, under certain conditions, to be simultaneous.' Suppose that I am simultaneously aware of a moving speck in the corner of my visual field and a slight tension in my left knee. Each of these is quite peripheral to my main object of attention, which is, say, a paper I am grading. I am not aware that I am aware of both of the peripheral events; and as in the previous case, such awareness may be impossible without losing the awareness of one of them. It may even be that my concentration on the paper is so intense that one or perhaps both of the peripheral events are lost to memory. Again, the three conscious events seem intuitively to belong to the same stream of consciousness; and one way of attempting to accommodate this is to weaken the necessary condition in the suggested way. The hope is that, were the attention directed to the paper less intense, the three conscious events would have been known, by either introspection or memory, to be simultaneous.

The merit of adopting either or both emendations is that there is less risk that normal people have, or appear to have, a disunified consciousness, while the behavior of split-brain subjects in the "key ring" experiments is still clear evidence for a disunified consciousness. But there are drawbacks as well. First, the inclusion of memory may make it impossible to decide whether these patients have a divided consciousness without first deciding how many subjects they contain. There are mechanisms for the exchange of information between disconnected hemispheres, e.g., cross-cuing. It is entirely likely that, after the "key ring" experiment is concluded and these mechanisms are allowed free rein, the split-brain patient may come to know that he saw both 'key' and 'ring' on the screen during the experiment. If this is memory knowledge, then he has, on the weaker criterion, a unified consciousness. If it is not to count as memory knowledge, the reason is presumably that the exchange of information between the disconnected hemispheres is akin to coming to know something on the basis of another's testimony. But how is this to be decided without first deciding whether there are two minds, giving testimony to each other? Second, the trouble with weakening 'known' to 'known, given certain conditions' is that there seems no principled way of excluding unfettered communications between the hemispheres as part of the conditions. And, of course, if this cannot be done, split-brain patients have a unified consciousness. The usual way that such conditions are specified is to point to some examples in which the subject has the requisite knowledge; the problem, in the present case, is that such examples are all cases in which, whatever other factors may be involved, the subject has unsevered commissures.

So I am inclined to let my necessary condition for unity of consciousness stand, and allow that our consciousness may be, on occasion, disunified. But I am not sure that the sort of examples I gave would show this. The one concerning memory is very hard to elaborate in a way that makes it clear that both events are conscious, and yet one is unaware that both events are occurring simultaneously. Even if that can be done, it is part of the example that the fact that both occurred simultaneously is immediately available to memory; and it might be that what we ordinarily call introspective knowledge is just this kind of memory knowledge, mediated, perhaps, by rapid shifts of attention. The problem with the second case, the one favoring weakening the knowledge condition, is similar. It is hard to elaborate in a way that makes it clear that one was consciously aware of *both* peripheral events, but the knowledge that both were occurring at the same time is unavailable to either memory or introspection. The clearer their unavailability, the more it looks as though the peripheral events were not consciously attended to.

IS THE CONSCIOUSNESS OF SPLIT-BRAIN
PATIENTS ALWAYS DISUNIFIED?

Split-brain patients sometimes have a disunified consciousness: that is, under certain experimental conditions, they have simultaneous conscious experiences whose joint occurrence is not introspectively disclosed. Is this disunity of consciousness confined to the experimental situation, or is it a standing condition? The usual answer is that split-brain patients always have a disunified consciousness, although this fact is masked by the integration of their everyday behavior. I want to contest this.

There are two positions which require somewhat different treatment. The first, held by Sperry and most neuropsychologists, is that split-brain patients always have a disunified consciousness but that people with commissures intact do not. The second, held by Puccetti, is that split-brain patients always have a disunified consciousness and so do we. I shall consider them in turn, concentrating on Sperry's.

The basic argument for Sperry's position is that the cause of the disunity in consciousness, behaviorally evident under experimental control, is the severing of the cerebral commissures, which remain severed when the split-brain patient leaves the laboratory. The problem is to explain the integration of his everyday behavior without implying that his consciousness is unified. Although cerebral dominance plays some role, the explanation relies primarily on two kinds of facts. First, information is *independently* duplicated in both hemispheres in a variety of ways, for example, by movements of sensory receptors, shared input from the face and neck, and ipsilateral feedback systems. Roughly, the mark of independent duplication of a bit of information is that there is no direct causal connection between its neural representation in one hemisphere and the corresponding representation in the other; rather there are separate causal paths, usually from sensory receptors, to each. Second, each hemisphere has some access to the contents of the

other through intact subcortical routes and, perhaps less importantly, through a variety of "cross-cuing" strategies.[31] In the experimental situation, where there are controls against independent
duplication and cross-cuing, the behavior of a split-brain patient
shows that his consciousness is disunified because the contents of
the two hemispheres differ in task-relevant ways. But, in everyday
circumstances, independent duplication of information, intact subcortical routes, and possibly cross-cuing strategies assure the same
task-relevant information in the two hemispheres; hence there is
no behavioral indication of disunity. Yet there is disunity, two
separate consciousnesses with largely overlapping contents rather
than a single unified consciousness, because the mechanisms which
serve to integrate behavior fail to unify consciousness. The factors
that contribute to independent duplication of information in the
hemispheres, while providing for similar contents, fail to provide
any access for one hemisphere to the contents of the other because the corresponding neural representations are achieved by
causally independent paths.[32] The intact subcortical routes are
not themselves powerful enough to unify consciousness, as is
shown in the experimental situation. And, finally, the cross-cuing
strategies do not differ in principle from the ways in which we
may come to know what someone else is experiencing.

A full and proper assessment of Sperry's position would require
reviewing a considerable amount of neurological and experimental
detail. But the situation can be outlined with the help of a few
broad distinctions. The mechanisms which contribute to the integration of behavior are divisible into two classes: commissural (the
commissures severed in Vogel and Bogen's version of commissurotomy) and extra-commissural (everything else). The corpus callosum is the prime example of the former; the various mechanisms
for independent duplication, subcortical paths between the hemispheres, and cross-cuing strategies are examples of the latter. The
extra-commissural mechanisms can themselves be divided into two
classes, those which independently duplicate information in the

hemispheres and those which, like subcortical paths and cross-cuing, involve direct causal connections between corresponding representations in the two hemispheres. With these distinctions in tow, the overall picture looks like this.[33]

(1) In the relevant experimental situations—where input is lateralized and there are controls against independent duplication of task-relevant information and cross-cuing—a split-brain subject's behavior is not integrated and he has a disunified consciousness. The only mechanisms available for behavioral integration are extra-commissural, excluding cross-cuing and independent duplication; and these fail.

(2) In similar experimental situations, a normal subject exhibits integrated behavior and has, on Sperry's view, a unified consciousness. The behavioral integration is achieved through commissural means.

(3) In everyday situations, where there are no controls on independent duplication or cross-cuing, the behavior of a normal subject is integrated; and he has, on Sperry's view, a unified consciousness. The mechanisms responsible for the integration are presumably both commissural and extra-commissural.

(4) In similar everyday situations, a split-brain patient exhibits integrated behavior,[34] achieved by extra-commissural mechanisms. The question is whether, as Sperry claims, he has a disunified consciousness.

The crucial issue is (a) whether independent duplication of information in the hemispheres serves to unify consciousness or (b) whether, in the absence of controls on independent duplication, the remaining direct neural connections between the hemispheres and, possibly, cross-cuing strategies serve to unify consciousness.

So there are two possible lines to pursue against Sperry. The more interesting, and radical, path is to claim that the independent duplication of information suffices for unity of consciousness. I think there are substantive philosophical considerations which favor this view; at a minimum, it runs little risk of direct empirical

refutation, since there is no serious behavioral evidence for disunity in consciousness unless the mechanisms for independent
duplication have been defeated. But, before considering what
favors this view, let us see what can be said against it.

An intuitive case against supposing that the mechanisms for independent duplication also serve to unify consciousness might run
as follows: Imagine that the "key ring" experiment is altered so
that 'key key,' instead of 'key ring,' is flashed on the screen. Although the split-brain subject will not correctly report what was
on the screen, there will be no behavior indicating a disunified
consciousness. Yet there is disunity, two seeings of 'key,' not one.
The environment has been manipulated to provide, by independent neural pathways, the same information to both sides of the
bisected brain. How could the presentation of 'key key' unify consciousness and that of 'key ring' divide it? Now consider what happens if 'key ring' is exposed long enough to allow eye movement.
The scanning movements of the eyes serve the same purpose as the
previous environmental duplication of 'key,' assuring, again via
separate neural pathways, that each hemisphere receives the information that 'key ring' was on the screen. How could such a duplication of information, achieved by relatively peripheral means,
unify consciousness while a more restricted view of the environment, as in the "key ring" experiment proper, divides it?[35] There
is still no access for one hemisphere to the contents of the other.
Even though both share a common environmental cause, the neural
representation of 'key ring' is just as causally isolated from its
counterpart as those of 'key' and 'ring' in the "key ring" experiment.

The argument just presented is a partial defense and deploy-
ment of Sperry's most explicit criterion for a unified consciousness, at least on one natural reading of the criterion.[36] In "Mental
Phenomena as Causal Determinants in Brain Function," he writes:

A cerebral process acts as a conscious entity, not because it is spatially set apart from other cerebral activity, but because it functions organizationally as a unit. . . . Normally, with the neocommissures intact, neural events in the right and left upper arms of our schematized Y substrate of consciousness become merged into a unified conscious brain process. The criterion for unity is an operational one; that is, the right and left components, coalesced through commissural connection, function in brain dynamics as a unit. This is illustrated in the unified visual perception of a stimulus figure flashed tachistoscopically half in the left and half in the right visual half-fields. In the normal brain the right and left hemispheric components combine and function as a unit in the causal sequence of cerebral control. In the divided brain, on the other hand, each hemisphere component gets its own separate causal effect as a distinct entity.[37]

The crucial notion of a unit is admittedly vague. But one relatively straightforward construal is that a brain process will function as a unit only if its components are causally connected in a fairly direct way, on some reasonable understanding of 'direct.' That is why the mental representations of 'key ring,' obtained by independent duplication, do not function as a unit and there are two conscious experiences, not one, even though they serve to integrate behavior. A set of neural events in the right and left hemispheres cannot be the physical basis of a single conscious experience unless they are themselves causally connected.

However persuasive it may appear, the argument against supposing that independent duplication unifies consciousness is far from secure. The following two cases should cause some doubts. (1) Given the available evidence,[38] it is probable that information transferred across the corpus callosum is largely redundant, at least from the standpoint of behavioral integration in normal circumstances. Imagine that, as seems possible, each hemisphere has a device that filters out the redundant signals so that they play no direct causal role in the integration of behavior. Then most of our behavioral integration would be largely the product of the same mechanisms for the independent duplication of information, which along with other factors, accounts for the normalcy of the split-brain patient's everyday behavior.[39] So it seems that, on Sperry's criterion, we *may* all have a disunified consciousness *most* of the time, although it is not shown in our behavior. (2) Imagine that we were so constructed that it was impossible to defeat the mechanisms for independent duplication; for example, our eyes might have moved too fast for tachistoscopic presentation to ensure lateralization of visual information in split-brain patients. If we were so constructed, there would be no possible behavioral evidence for a disunified consciousness in split-brain patients. Is it obvious that commissurotomy would then produce permanent undetectable disunity in consciousness, as Sperry must claim, rather than none at all?

These doubts derive from the reasonable principle that the sort of behavioral integration we exhibit, and which split-brain patients exhibit outside the experimental situation, is very strong prima facie evidence for unity of consciousness. The claim that split-brain patients usually have a consciousness unified by the mechanisms for independent duplication respects the presumption the behavior creates. Moreover, it is a simpler hypothesis than the rival claim that split-brain patients always have a disunified consciousness. Split-brain patients are very much like us behaviorally. If we account for our integrated behavior, at least in part, by assuming unity of consciousness and can do the same for split-brain patients, why not do so? Then the moral of experiments like the "key ring" experiment is that bilateral neural representation is a physical basis for unity of consciousness; but it is irrelevant how such representation is achieved, whether through the commissures or through mechanisms for independent duplication. Disunity in consciousness is still available *precisely* where it is needed: to explain the abnormal behavior of split-brain patients in the experiments. The disunity is itself explained by the fact that the experimental controls defeat the mechanisms which are, as a result of commissurotomy, responsible for unity of consciousness in these patients. Similarly there is a natural explanation for the behavioral differences between split-brain patients and normal controls. The mechanisms which subserve unity of consciousness in the normal controls differ in ways that make them immune to failure in the experimental situation.[40]

Freed from question-begging associations, the case against the independent duplication of information unifying consciousness is not powerful enough to override the behavioral evidence. Talk of the lack of information exchange or communication between the disconnected hemispheres invites us to portray the two hemispheres as subjects of experience or minds.[41] If we do, the case against independent duplication seems obvious: in the absence of direct causal connection, one mind cannot have access to the other's experience in the way it has access to its own. But the number of minds a split-brain patient has is just what is at issue. Apart from the question-begging associations, the crucial causal principle is not strongly motivated.[42] Why should neural processes unrelated by direct causal routes not be the physical basis for a single mental state? If one accepts—as I do—the general account of mind advocated by philosophers as diverse as Fodor[43] and Grice,[44] there is some reason for thinking they sometimes are. On this view, minds are the things which have mental states; and mental states are the states required by an adequate psychological theory of the organism.[45] This account does not require corresponding types of neurological states for each type of psychological state. Nor does it require any direct causal links between the neural events which are the physical basis for a single psychological state. It would be sufficient if causally unrelated neural events jointly, though separately, produced effects which were, from the standpoint of the psychology, the basis of a single mental state. Since it is a commonplace that the neurological structure of human brain is highly redundant, as might be expected of a biologically viable system, it should not be surprising if the redundancy is sometimes irrelevant for the purposes of psychology. Of course, it is an empirical question whether an adequate psychology will construe the dual neural representations caused by independent duplication in split-brain patients as single psychological states; but there is no reason in principle against doing so.

However the issue of divided consciousness is settled, no amount of reconstruction will save Sperry's criterion when it comes to deciding how many minds or conscious subjects there are in split-brain subjects. The ambient visual field of the split-brain patient is unified even in the experimental setup.[46] Thus, for example, if a moving spot is flashed in the periphery of the left visual field, the split-brain patient can both report the fact and indicate, left-handed, a similar awareness. Presumably this is accounted for by subcortical structures. On Sperry's (and any reasonable) criterion, there is a single experience of seeing the spot. Call this experience A. While the spot is flashed, two different odors or sounds may be presented, one to the left, the other to the right hemisphere. Call the associated experiences B and C. B and C are distinct experiences by Sperry's (and any reasonable) criterion. What mind, conscious entity, conscious subject, or whatever has the experiences?[47] Sperry contends that distinct minds, say LB and RB, have B and C. Who or what has A? Not both, for there is a single experience. Not LB rather than RB, or vice versa, for that is incompatible with the behavioral evidence. So either there is a *third* mind which has A, which, at a minimum, is incompatible with the two-minds account or, more plausibly, there are really two distinct A-like experiences, which is incompatible with the criterion. And the criterion cannot be lightly abandoned. For, if it is, we have disunity in consciousness, two distinct A-like experiences, when there are direct neural connections between the representations in the two hemispheres and there is no behavioral evidence of disunity. So why is *our* consciousness not always disunified?

The other possible line against Sperry is that cross-cuing strategies and the remaining direct neural connections between the separated hemispheres, e.g., subcortical routes, serve to unify the consciousness of split-brain patients outside the experimental situation. This line of attack has many of the virtues of the previous one and some of its own as well. One need not question in any wholesale way the crucial assumption that unity of consciousness requires direct causal connections between the corresponding representations in the left and right hemispheres. But the dialectical advantages of conservatism are bought, as we shall shortly see, by assuming a considerable empirical debt. The price may or may not be prohibitive.

There are two basic points against this position. First, the exchange of information via cross-cuing strategies is incompatible with the supposition of a unified consciousness, since such strategies do not differ in principle from the ways in which two separate minds acquire information about each other. Second, the split-brain experiments show that the remaining direct neural connections are not powerful enough to unify consciousness when cross-cuing and the independent duplication of information are controlled against.

The first point can be met. The reason cross-cuing seems incompatible with unity of consciousness is that it is taken to involve a primitive intentional exchange of information and, as such, to require two minds to conduct the exchange.[48] But there is no convincing evidence for an intentional exchange of information between the disconnected hemispheres; and the usual claim that the alleged two minds are unaware of each other's existence directly contradicts such an assumption.[49] The exchange of information by cross-cuing appears to be as unintended and unconscious as the flow of information across the corpus callosum. So it seems possible to view cross-cuing simply as an exchange of information between the hemispheres by peripheral routes, which, like the exchange conducted through the commissures, is neutral on the two-minds question.

The second point creates a serious problem. The view in question is, in effect, that under the conditions which obtain when there are no controls on the mechanisms for independent duplication, the remaining neural connections and cross-cuing unify the consciousness of split-brain patients. So someone favoring this view is forced to explain why, in the absence of independent duplication and cross-cuing, the remaining, presumably subcortical, neural connections fail to unify consciousness. This is a fair burden and not one easily discharged. For example, one cannot exploit the relatively short exposure times of visual stimuli like those in the "key ring" experiment because other modalities, e.g., stereognosis, allow for much longer exposure times. And, even in the case of vision, it is now possible, thanks to Zaidel's occluders,[50] to allow exposure times up to one half hour and still elicit the same kind of behavioral evidence for disunity.

On the other hand, there are some empirical grounds for modest optimism. Unity of consciousness can be achieved with considerably *fewer* than the tremendous number of neural connections furnished by the intact commissures, even when information is not independently duplicated in the hemispheres. There are cases of total asymptomatic agenesis of the corpus callosum, that is, of people who are born without a corpus callosum and exhibit no symptoms. By itself, this is not remarkable in light of the normal behavior of split-brain patients in everyday situations and the plasticity of the developing nervous system. What is remarkable is that such agenesis subjects behave like normal controls when subjected to the same experimental tests as split-brain patients.[51] Sperry writes:

> This 19-year-old college sophomore, with an average scholastic record and previously presumed to be normal until hospitalized and x-rayed for a series of headaches, easily went through the entire battery of cross-integration tests we had devised for the surgical patients, performing essentially like a normal control subject. Even words projected half to one and half to the other hemisphere, near the threshold of visual acuity, were read off promptly with no difficulty. This was true even when the pronunciation depended upon the two halves of the word.[52]

Since her behavior does not differ from ours in any relevant respects under any conditions, I assume that Sperry would agree that she has a unified consciousness and, so, that the presence of the corpus callosum is not required for unity of consciousness. But, although they lack a corpus callosum, agenesis subjects retain other minor commissures which are severed in the kind of commissurotomy performed by Vogel and Bogen, and these commissures are presumed to have developed abnormally. The contribution of the neural connections, which remain intact in split-brain patients, and cross-cuing to the integrated behavior of agenesis subjects is unknown. Results obtained from testing a commissurotomy patient in whom the anterior commissure was spared point in the same direction.[53] In this case, there was an extensive preoperative as well as postoperative assessment of cognitive function. On all tests, including some involving tachistoscopic presentation, he improved postoperatively. But, again, this patient retained a minor commissure which is severed by Vogel and Bogen; and it is not known how cross-cuing and the neural connections left intact by Vogel and Bogen contribute to the integration of his behavior. Perhaps the later performance of one of Bogen's patients is more to the point. Seven years after the operation, L. B. was able to read across midline, although not as well as a normal control.[54] Since he was a patient of Bogen's, the mechanisms must be entirely extra-commissural. So there is some evidence that, as far as some visual processes are concerned, the extra-commissural system may have the *potential* to unify consciousness, even under conditions which formerly elicited behavioral evidence of disunity.

The above may seem like small consolation. Even if the extra-commissural system has the potential to unify the consciousness of split-brain patients, why does it fail to do so under the experimental controls and not in everyday life? In lieu of any plausible candidate explanation, the advantage would definitely be Sperry's—other things being equal. But Sperry has a considerable empirical burden of his own. On his view, unity of consciousness is irrelevant to behavioral integration (and to most cognitive functions so far as they are evident in behavior) in all but the most artificial circumstances. On normal and natural assumptions about the contribution of unity of consciousness to integrated action, this is surely surprising and in need of explanation. If no explanation is possible, the presumption is that other extra-commissural mechanisms serve to unify consciousness. On the other hand, if there is an explanation of how such thoroughgoing behavioral integration can be achieved without unity of consciousness, it is no longer clear that unity of consciousness bears upon unity of mind in the way we normally assume. For, given the efficient cognitive functioning of split-brain patients and their usually integrated behavior, it no longer seems impossible to maintain that they have a single mind, even though it is characterized by the kind of totally disunified consciousness Sperry attributes to these patients.[55] I would not have to be much of a skeptic to convince myself that I may have a totally disunified consciousness of this sort; the conviction that I may have two minds is a lot harder to come by. Thus, as matters now stand, the conservative line, as well as the radical one, are viable unrefuted alternatives to Sperry's position.

Puccetti's version of the thesis that split-brain patients always have a disunified consciousness remains to be considered. Since Puccetti denies that a normal, commissure-intact human being has a unified consciousness and a single mind, his position requires, at least in part, separate treatment. The quickest way is to show that he is not entitled to separate treatment. Although it is less explicit and differs in some details, Puccetti's argument that we all have two minds (and are two persons) parallels the one sketched on pp. 6–10.[56] He proceeds from earlier conclusions that split-brain patients lack unity of consciousness, have two minds, and are two persons to similar claims about us. And he intends to do so, so far as I can tell, by an argument like the one I offered on pp. 9–10 to justify the step from (4) to (5): that the best explanation of how there are two minds or persons in split-brain patients after the operation requires two before as well.[57] But that argument is defective, and so Puccetti's position does not need separate treatment. The explanation of how there can be two minds after the operation requires only that there be, before the operation, a single mind which is potentially, not actually, two. Given natural assumptions, it is enough that the single mind have a highly redundant physical basis or one that allows for suitable reorganization or both. One may be, though I even doubt this, forced to maintain that both the resulting minds are new. But, so long as talk of communication between the hemispheres via the commissures is not taken to imply that before the operation each hemisphere had conscious experiences of which the other was kept informed,[58] there is no reason to suppose that there must be two minds before the operation if there are two afterward.[59]

Quite independently, Puccetti's position faces some severe epistemological difficulties. If one were convinced that split-brain patients always have a disunified consciousness, his position would be a natural outcome of the previous criticism of Sperry: that, as far as unity of consciousness is concerned, there is no relevant difference between bilateral representation obtained through the commissures or by extra-commissural means. So, if split-brain patients always have a divided consciousness, we do too. The problem is why one should be convinced that they do. For both Sperry and Puccetti, the initial evidence for a split in the consciousness of split-brain patients is their behavior in the experimental situation. Sperry appeals to an anatomical difference between split-brain patients and normal controls to justify his claim that the consciousness of split-brain patients is always disunified; and the appeal is plausible because the difference explains why split-brain patients behave abnormally in the experimental situation and why normal controls do not. But no such appeal is available to Puccetti since, on his view, both split-brain patients and normal controls always lack unity of consciousness, despite their neurological and behavioral differences. His position can be maintained only by identifying some factor, shared by us and split-brain patients, which is responsible for the disunity; and the only candidate, as far as I can tell, is the stark fact that, both in us and in split-brain patients, information, sometimes the same information, receives a neural representation in both hemispheres. But normal, commissure-intact individuals have such dual representation in the total absence of behavior indicative of disunity of consciousness.[60] So one needs an argument that bilateral representation, all by itself, suffices for disunity. The prospects look dim.[61]

CAN A SINGLE MIND EVER HAVE A DISUNIFIED CONSCIOUSNESS?

Thus far, I have argued that, although the consciousness of split-brain subjects is disunified under experimental conditions, there is no compelling reason to think that it is disunified otherwise. Of course, if a single mind could not tolerate even occasional lapses in the unity of consciousness, the experimental data would implicate two minds for split-brain patients and dictate an explanation of the normalcy of their behavior outside the experimental situation in terms of communication between the two minds. No doubt, most of the minds we are acquainted with have unified consciousness; and we do believe that the conscious contents of a single mind at a given moment occur in a unified stream of consciousness. But that does not prejudice the issue of whether the split-brain cases show this belief to be false, rather than the belief dictating a two-minds account.

I read Nagel[62] as claiming that it is impossible, given our ordinary unanalyzed concept of mind, that a single mind *ever* can have a consciousness disunified in the way the split-brain patient's is in the "key-ring" experiment. In *Brain Bisection and the Unity of Consciousness,* he seeks to establish that the split-brain studies show that our idea of the unity of a person cannot be coordinated with an understanding of human beings as physical systems; and an essential step is to show that there is no whole number of minds split-brain patients have. Nagel's argument that they do not have one mind runs as follows:

> For in these patients there appear to be things happening simultaneously which cannot fit into a single mind . . . . Lack of interaction in the domain of visual experience threatens assumptions about the unity of consciousness which are basic to our understanding of another individual as a person . . . . These assumptions . . . make it impossible to arrive at an interpretation of the cases under discussion in terms of a countable number of minds . . . . Roughly, we assume that a single mind has sufficiently immediate access to its conscious states so that, for elements of experience or other mental events occurring simultaneously or in close temporal proximity, the mind which is their subject can also experience the simpler *relations* between them if it attends to the matter . . . . Split-brain patients fail dramatically to conform to these assumptions in experimental situations, and they fail over the simplest matters.[63]

A few pages later, he concludes that "the fundamental problem in trying to understand these cases in mentalistic terms is that we take ourselves as paradigms of mental unity, and are then unable to project ourselves into their mental lives either once or twice".[64] As I understand it, the assumptions "basic to our understanding of another individual as a person" are supposed to imply that a single mind could never have the kind of disunity of consciousness exhibited by split-brain patients in experiments like the "key ring" experiment; and this is supposed to be a consequence of our intuitive, unanalyzed understanding of the concept of mind.

I think that this is incorrect. Consider the following case. It is now possible, using the techniques pioneered by Wada,[65] to anesthetize the cerebral hemispheres selectively. Although it is not now possible to anesthetize the cerebral commissures selectively, it is easy enough to imagine this being done. Suppose my corpus callosum and the other minor commissures were selectively anesthetized for, say, ten minutes. If I were a subject in the "key ring" experiments, I would behave just like the split-brain patients. There would be the same behavioral evidence for a disunified consciousness, implying for the time I was anesthetized, a separation of conscious mental phenomena exactly analogous to that of split-brain patients. Moreover, the conscious mental states associated with each hemisphere would have the same kind of internal coherence as those of the split-brain patients. I doubt that the ordinary conception of mind requires any description of this case other than that I, for ten minutes, had a disunified consciousness.[66] To think otherwise immediately buys a lot of theoretical trouble. If, for example, I had two minds during the interval, was one or both new, and is the mind that existed before I was anesthetized the same as the one that exists afterward? These questions *may* be answerable, but I do not see that we are forced, in virtue of our shared concept of mind, to raise them.

I also think Nagel is wrong in thinking that the fundamental problem in trying to understand split-brain patients is our inability to project ourselves into their mental lives, either once or twice. This diagnosis assumes the sort of account of understanding another he later amplifies in *What Is It Like to Be a Bat?*[67] I am generally sympathetic to that account; but, even if understanding the mental life of another requires knowing what it is like to be the other and one way we do this is to project ourselves imaginatively into the other's consciousness, it is not relevant to the split-brain phenomena. For there is nothing special "it is like" to be a split-brain patient. Whatever dissociation of consciousness a split-brain patient endures is not, nor could it be, a fact introspectively disclosed.[68] The limits of projection are just that we cannot imagine that we have a disunified consciousness and, at the same time, introspect all its contents; but neither can the split-brain patient.

SOME ROUGH TRUTH CONDITIONS FOR 'SPLIT-BRAIN PATIENTS HAVE ONE (TWO) MIND(S)'

The result of the preceding two sections is that there is no compelling reason to think that split-brain patients always have a divided consciousness or that a single mind can never have the kind of disunified consciousness the split-brain patients exhibit under experimental situations. Although this seriously weakens the case for a two-minds account, it leaves the principal question unanswered: can a single mind have both the kind and number of lapses in the unity of consciousness endured by split-brain patients? Until now, I have relied mainly, as most of the literature does, on our intuitive understanding of the concept of mind. This is no longer possible because our question cannot be answered without some principled way of determining how disunity in consciousness bears upon unity of mind. And I cannot see how this could be done without something like relevant truth conditions for these patients having one or two minds. So we need enough of a theory of mind to suggest and motivate the truth conditions.

As I mentioned earlier, I accept, in broad outline, the sort of account of mind offered by philosophers as different as Fodor, Grice, and Perry.[69] The heart of that account is that 'mind' and mental concepts are part of a theory intended, *inter alia*, to explain behavior. We all know a lot, however rough, inexact, and hedged, about how human beings behave. Part of what we know has a wider scope, applying, say, to any material body. But a great deal of what we know applies primarily to the behavior of human beings or closely related species. Perry calls this the "human theory" and gives, as examples, our knowledge that "if we ask a human being if he would like his toe stepped on, he will probably say 'no'; that when deprived of food for a long time, he will probably seek it; that shortly after observing something with care he will be able to recall what he observed; and so forth."[70] We think we can explain why the propositions about human behavior, which constitute the "human theory," hold. Our explanations rely on a network of interacting internal states, which are largely, but not exclusively, specified by our names for propositional attitudes, e.g., memory, belief, desire, intention. The tacit understanding we have of their interaction and their contribution to behavior constitutes our folk psychology; and it is regularly deployed in our everyday explanations of human behavior in terms of propositional attitudes. We think, for example, that what a human being does in a choice situation is a function of how he views the situation, what he takes his behavioral options and their consequences to be, and how he ranks the consequences. Thus, it is because, among other things, a human being assigns a relatively low value to having his toes squashed, given the option of having them left alone, that he says 'no' when asked whether he would like his toes stepped on. Like the knowledge it explains, folk psychology is inexact, hedged by "usually's," "probably's," and "*ceteris paribus*'s"; and the efficacy of the rough and ready explanations it licenses is itself explicable. Our commonsense psychology has some purchase on a finer structure of internal events, states, and processes which will explain why people have the thoughts, beliefs, wants, intentions, and so forth that the folk psychology attributes to them. My belief is that it is the aim of a scientific psychology to characterize this structure. Thus, for example, I think of a psychologist's account of memory—with its distinctions between sensory store, short-, and long-term memory, specifications of how information is encoded, stored, and retrieved, etc.—as an attempt to characterize the finer structure of internal events and processes that warrant our everyday explanations of behavior in terms of someone's remembering this or that. Similarly, I view learning theory and theories of development as providing refined accounts of certain kinds of transitions between the inner states.

So I think human minds are those entities the states of which explain our propositional attitudes and, by extension, explain why our everyday mentalistic explanations of human behavior are approximately correct. And I expect the account of the relevant states and transitions between them to be furnished by a true, adequate psychology for human beings. If mind is understood in this way, the natural suggestion is that whether split-brain patients have one mind or two is a matter of whether the most satisfactory explanations of their behavior come from a single or double application of a true, adequate psychological theory for human beings. Or put another way, it is a matter of whether each hemisphere of these patients, or their entire brain, is the best candidate for having the states the true human psychology countenances.

HOW DOES DISUNITY OF CONSCIOUSNESS BEAR UPON UNITY OF MIND?

In light of the previous section, the answer is: only insofar as it forces a double, rather than a single, application of a correct psychology in order to get satisfactory explanations of behavior. Whatever its defects, this answer has one immediate virtue. It seems unlikely that an adequate psychology will insist that all or most mental phenomena are conscious, and it seems equally unlikely that it will endorse the Cartesian claim that minds are somehow transparent to their possessors. So there is room to ask how disunity of consciousness, of various kinds and degrees, will disrupt the explanations the psychology endorses. Disruption is a matter of degree, and there is no reason to think that every kind and degree of disunity will require such radical measures as supposing that the subject has two minds.[71]

The big drawback, of course, is that we do not have a true adequate psychology for human beings. Indeed, since we do not, it may even seem strange that we believe normal human beings have a single mind if the account of mind I have endorsed is true. But it is not so strange if folk psychology is cast in the role of the

unknown true scientific psychology. I am inclined to think that
our belief that minds come one to a body is due to the fact that,
in explaining the behavior of human beings, our ordinary explanatory schemata—such as the explanation of choice behavior in
terms of belief and desire—require only a single, relatively stable,
and comprehensibly changeable structure of propositional attitudes. The notion of such a structure of propositional attitudes is
vague, but the idea will become clearer by considering a situation
in which it is clearly absent. If I am right, we should be inclined to
describe it, with minimal discomfort, as a case of two minds in
one body. The case is that of Mary Reynolds, a classic of multiple
personality. Sutcliffe and Jones present the following summary of
her case history:

> Miss Reynolds was born in 1793, and died in 1854. Her disorder was
> first noticed at the age of 18 (1811). Before her alterations she was de-
> scribed as a well-educated young woman, of dull and melancholy tem-
> perament, living in the wilds of Pennsylvania. Her personality changed
> following a long and profound sleep. She awoke disoriented, no longer
> able to recognize relatives and unable to perform such learned skills as
> reading and writing. Previously reserved, taciturn and timid, she was
> now friendly, merry and adventurous, with a new interest in the out-
> doors. There was no regaining of self-reference memories, or reestab-
> lishment of old personal relationships in the "second state." However,
> retraining in reading and writing proceeded rapidly. After five weeks in
> State 2, on this first occasion, Miss R. returned to her old state (State
> 1), following a further profound sleep. Now, in State 1, there was no
> memory for the intervening State 2 period. Alternations between these
> two mutually amnesic phases went on for 15/16 years. Memory was
> continuous within each of the phases. Stabilization in a modified State
> 2 took place around age 35. Miss R. died suddenly, at age 61, complain-
> ing of a sudden strange sensation in the head. For the last 25 years of
> her life she remained in State 2.[72]

If we want to explain the actions of Mary Reynolds in State 1,
we appeal to sets of propositional attitudes, many of them standing beliefs and long-term wants and desires, which exclude, and
must exclude, a large number of the propositional attitudes we

need to explain her State 2 behavior. Thus, for example, part of the explanation of why Mary, in State 1, does not go for a romp through the woods on a pleasant afternoon is that she believes she has a duty toward her parents to do her assigned household chores. And part of the explanation of why Mary, in State 2, does not forgo the romp is that she does not even believe that those people are her parents and hence does not believe that she is under any particular obligation to tend their house. The successive sets of propositional attitudes we use to explain her State 1 behavior have a familiar kind of internal coherence, and they follow each other, with various changes and overlaps, in the way we expect; and those for State 2 do so as well. Each, separately, looks like part of a typical psychological history of a single person. But if we attempt to combine them, that is, take the successive sets of propositional attitudes in their true temporal order, we can maintain the internal coherence of the individual sets on each side of a transition between State 1 and State 2 only by making it unintelligible how they could be parts of the psychological history of a single person. On the other hand, if we take the successive sets of propositional attitudes associated with State 1 and those associated with State 2 as parts of the psychological histories of two persons, we can explain the behavior of each within a single, relatively stable, and comprehensibly changeable structure of propositional attitudes. That is why we are inclined to think Mary Reynolds is really two. A lot of analytic work would be required to specify what makes a given set of propositional attitudes "internally coherent" and a succeeding set "comprehensibly changeable"; but, in what follows, I rely only on some intuitive minimal conditions.

The case of Mary Reynolds is unlike that of the split-brain patients in that it does not involve any disunity of consciousness (and, of course, the two minds alternate temporally). Nonetheless, if my diagnosis of why we are inclined to think that Mary Reynolds had two minds is correct, we can distinguish our knowledge of unity of mind from our knowledge of unity of consciousness.

And we can see why a *massive* breakdown of unity of consciousness would lead us to talk of two minds: our ordinary explanations of the behavior of human beings in terms of a single structure of propositional attitudes could not survive such a breakdown. Assume that the conscious mental experiences of a subject are not jointly introspectible, not jointly available to memory, and differ in content. Assume also that such experiences have the usual relation to the subject's propositional attitudes, his beliefs, wants, memories, etc., and that his propositional attitudes are productive in the usual way. This kind of failure of unity of consciousness would completely disrupt our everyday explanations in terms of a single structure of beliefs, desires, memories, etc. Our usual grounds for attributing unity of mind to such an individual disappear completely. If we want to explain his behavior at all, we are forced to appeal to two different structures of propositional attitudes and, thus, to consider him as having two minds.

Split-brain patients do not exhibit such a massive breakdown in unity of consciousness, and the usual explanations in terms of propositional attitudes work as well for their everyday behavior as for ours. But these explanations do fail in situations like the "key ring" experiment, and they fail dramatically.[73] The split-brain subject points to 'key' because, among other things, he wants to cooperate with the experimenter by indicating what he saw and he believes he saw 'key.' Similarly, he says "ring" because he saw 'ring' and wants to indicate what he saw. So far, there is no difficulty. The trouble arises when we ask why he did not point to 'ring' or say "key." In order to explain this, it looks as though we must assume that he does not believe he saw 'ring' and he does not believe he saw 'key.'[74] But both the belief that he saw 'ring' and its absence cannot be attributed to a single mind or subject. Hence there must be two. This is an argument that split-brain patients have two minds which does not rely upon any facts about the consciousness of split-brain patients. We cannot apply our usual explanations of action in terms of belief and desire once. So we are tempted to apply them twice and, as a result, think that we must be dealing with two minds.

However tempting, the argument is defective. The utility of our usual explanations depends upon our being able, in general, to infer that someone does not believe *p* from his believing *not-p* and to infer that he does not believe *not-p* from his believing *p*. Normally this assumption is safe for uncomplicated perceptual judgments such as that one sees 'key' or not. But it fails for the split-brain patients in the experimental situation.[75] Its failure, however, admits of a straightforward explanation: split-brain patients, unlike us, have on occasion a disunified consciousness. That they have a disunified consciousness is, in turn, explained by the fact that the physical basis of their unity of consciousness is different from ours and, thus, liable to failure in situations where ours is not. The explanations of behavior our folk psychology licenses are crude. As such, they will tolerate the occasional failures the split-brain patients provide without recourse to such drastic measures as the supposition that they have two minds, and they will tolerate them easily if there is a readily available account of why they fail. The crucial fact is that our ordinary explanations fail only when different input is provided to each hemisphere, the input is of a sort that can be attended to by both hemispheres and differentially responded to, and no integration is possible by extra-commissural means. These conditions are highly artificial; a normal environment does not provide them. So our ordinary explanations of behavior usually work for split-brain patients. We need only admit their occasional failure, accounting for it in terms of a disunified consciousness, itself the product of a surgically induced anatomical difference between split-brain patients and us.

Even if folk psychology is taken to be the final word, it is logically possible that split-brain patients come to have two minds. If the environment provided (or were made to provide) different lateralized input beyond anything now possible, if divided attention were generally possible, and if the extra-commissural exchange of information between, or the duplication of it in, the hemispheres were limited in ways that now seem unlikely, then, perhaps, we would always have to apply our usual explanations of behavior to the split-brain subjects twice. But, on empirical grounds, it is unlikely that these conditions can be satisfied; and, I suppose, on ethical grounds, we should not attempt to. The empirical grounds are (1) that such lateralization of input is unlikely for an ambient human being in a relatively stable environment and (2) it would require that attentional mechanisms be divided to an extent not yet shown to be possible.[76]

WILL AN ADEQUATE PSYCHOLOGY FAVOR A ONE-MIND ACCOUNT OF SPLIT-BRAIN PATIENTS?

In the previous section, I sketched how disunity of consciousness bears upon unity of mind if our folk psychology and the explanatory schemata it employs are cast in the role of an adequate scientific psychology. Although a single mind could not have a massively disunified consciousness, it could endure the kind of disunity exhibited by the split-brain patients. However, in my view, the issue really turns on whether an adequate scientific psychology could tolerate the kind of disunified consciousness split-brain patients have. If the best explanation of the behavior of split-brain patients involves applying the psychological theory separately to each brain half, then they have two minds. Strictly speaking, the issue is undecidable in the absence of the psychology. But, given a few broad assumptions about what the psychology will be like, there is reason to bet that it will favor a one-mind account.

I assume that an adequate psychology will be of the information-processing sort, relying largely on the organism's handling of the information at its disposal to provide the raw material for psychological explanation. So the organism's various relations to internal representations, which encode the information at its disposal in one or more "languages of thought," will be central to the psychology. I also assume that, for the reasons adduced by Fodor,[77] there will be no possibility of reducing the psychological theory to a neurophysiological one. Finally, I assume that, from the standpoint of the psychology, the physical bases of at least some, and probably many, psychological states and processes will be redundant. That is, for a given psychological state, there will often be more than one physiological state which is sufficient for that psychological state; and the redundancy will not be psychologically relevant. This is presumably the case for many of the psychological states we now attribute, e.g., having a visual percept of 'key.'

Given these assumptions, the case that an adequate psychology will favor a one-mind account of split-brain patients runs as follows: We believe that unity of consciousness is at least part of the explanation of the behavioral integration exhibited by normal human beings. Either that belief is approximately correct or it is not. Suppose that it is. Since the psychology will also have to explain behavioral integration, one would expect it to contain a concept or set of concepts which is the scientific replacement for unity of consciousness. The heir of unity of consciousness would play a roughly similar role in explaining the behavioral integration of normal human beings. Since, apart from the experiments, the split-brain patients exhibit the same degree of behavioral integration we do, one would like to explain it in the same way, by appealing to the scientific successor of unity of consciousness. And, if this can be done, there will be no reason not to attribute the same unitary psychological states and processes to both split-brain patients and normals, although they will sometimes have a partially different physical basis in split-brain patients. The problem, of course, is the abnormal behavior of split-brain patients in the experimental situation. But it should be open to the psychology, just as it is open to our folk psychology, to attribute the abnormal behavior to the split-brain patient's temporary lack of whatever it is that replaces unity of consciousness. This in turn is to be explained by the fact that the neural mechanisms which subserve the replacement for unity of consciousness are different and thus subject to failure in the experimental conditions. This line, as opposed to treating each brain-half as a psychological subject, has the advantage of making the integrated action of both split-brain patients and us depend upon the same thing, the scientific successor of unity of consciousness. The appeal to disunity, or rather its heir, will be limited to those spots where it does some genuine work, namely, to where it explains a lack of behavioral integration. So there will be considerable pressure on the psychology to give a one-mind account of split-brain patients.

If we are grossly wrong in thinking that unity of consciousness is at least part of the explanation for our usual behavioral integration, the case is still much the same. There will still be a large incentive to explain the integration of the split-brain patient's everyday behavior in terms of the same psychological states and processes which explain ours. And, again, it seems that this will be possible if one allows that some of these states and processes have a somewhat different physical basis in split-brain patients. The difference in physical basis will, as before, provide the explanation of their lack of integrated behavior in the experimental situation. So again it seems unlikely that the best explanation of the split-brain patient's behavior will require treating each brain-half as a psychological subject. The only difference, as far as I can see, will be in what we may be willing to say about unity of consciousness. In the event that unity of consciousness turns out to be a mere epiphenomenon, one would not expect the psychology to contain any replacing concept; and unity of consciousness as such will be irrelevant to unity of mind. So it would not matter much what we say about the unity or disunity of the split-brain patient's consciousness. But then what we say about our own unity or disunity of consciousness would not matter either.

Whether split-brain patients have one mind or two is, in the long run, an empirical issue, although it will not be decided by the experiments currently being done.[78] I do not think that there are any logical grounds for rejecting a two-minds account of split-brain patients. After all, attempts to explain the behavior and cognition of normal human beings in terms of more than one mind, or in terms of mind parts, are as old as Plato.[79] Such accounts are usually motivated by conflicts, whether conflicts in desire, or belief, or action. The fundamental move is to apportion the conflicting desires, beliefs, or actions to minds or mind-parts which are themselves conflict-free. The structural richness and capabilities of the minds or mind-parts are determined by the number of mental processes or possibilities of behavior implicated by the conflicting phenomena. The distinction between whole minds and mind-parts is artificial. It tends to collapse as the mind-parts are assigned wider ranges of mental functions and are allowed to control wider ranges of the organism's behavior. The usual trouble with accounts which rely on psychic fission is their explanatory adequacy. To the extent that the independent minds or quasi-minds have differing structures of wants and beliefs, our usual degree of integration is a puzzle. To the extent that they have a common set of wants and beliefs, they seem extravagant. I suspect that, *mutatis mutandis,* this is the problem a two-minds account of split-brain patients faces; and I have speculated that an adequate psychology will avoid, as our commonsense psychology can, the extravagance.

WITTGENSTEINIAN POSTSCRIPT

Philosophical problems often arise, Wittgenstein maintained, because we have crude, but compelling, ways of representing complex phenomena. A particular picture, reinforced by the anatomy of the human brain, causes a great deal of mischief in thinking about split-brain phenomena. The picture is that of the two hemispheres exchanging information, communicating, or even "talking" with each other via the corpus callosum. Suppose that one starts with the commonsense view that our consciousnesses are unified. It is natural to interpret the split-brain experiments as showing that our unity of consciousness is the product of the communication between the hemispheres effected by the corpus callosum and other commissures. If the commissures are severed, there are two noncommunicating centers of consciousness, however similar their contents may be. Whatever noncommissural mechanisms serve to duplicate content in the disconnected hemispheres cannot unify consciousness because they do not provide the kind of communication between the hemispheres that the commissures do. And that kind of communication, as the experiments seem to show, is essential to unity of consciousness. It is but a short step from here to the standard view that split-brain patients, unlike us, have two minds. On the other hand, if one begins by focusing on the fact that the hemispheres *communicate* by means of the corpus callosum, the outcome is different. It is natural to think of this as one hemisphere's being made aware of the experiences of the other and perhaps even being brought to have similar experiences as well. The split-brain operation disrupts the lines of communication and so enables us to *discover* that there were two conscious subjects all along. Thus we have the incredible view that we all have two minds, although this fact is usually masked by the rapid access they have to each other's contents. Whichever way the picture leads, it is abetted by our cerebral anatomy. If, while looking at a schematic drawing of the brain, one imagines the commissures, those lines of communication between the hemispheres, severed, one can almost *see* how many minds there are—or so it seems.

A major part of the trouble is that we do not, as yet, have a philosophically satisfying account of what is meant by statements like 'The hemispheres exchange information, or communicate, via the corpus callosum.' Clearly more is involved than the fact that neural events originating in one hemisphere have, by way of the corpus callosum, effects in the other; and part of what is involved is that the neural events transmit a message encoded in something like a language. It is only very recently that philosophers have begun to provide general accounts of what it is for physical events, other than tokens of the sentences we use to communicate with each other, to encode information. But, whatever the proper account is, it cannot require construing the exchange of information between the hemispheres on the model of two people talking to one another because the exchange of information via the commissures does not differ in principle from other neural exchanges of information within the hemispheres. Presumably, no one thinks that each hemisphere decomposes into still more conscious subjects or minds.

In the final analysis, pictures are not argued against but are replaced by others we hope are less misleading on the matters at issue. The picture that underlies this work is that we and the split-brain patients are basically the same kinds of psychological devices, although our hardware is somewhat different. Under most conditions, we and the split-brain patients perform similarly; in some comparatively rare and highly artificial environmental conditions, the hardware differences come into play. However, the fact that the mechanisms they have available to unify consciousness sometimes fail does not mean that they do not work at all or that they do not normally serve the same purposes ours do. This, too, is only a picture, crude and misleading in its own way; but, if the arguments of this monograph are correct, it is less misleading on the number of minds split-brain patients have.

NOTES

1. See the bibliography. Although it contains a fair number of such studies, they are just a selection from a much larger literature. For example, at least 80 articles dealing in some measure with the psychological effects of commissurotomy were published in medical and psychological journals between January 1977 and June 1978. I have included papers which, for a variety of reasons, I thought relevant to this work. I think Bogen (1969a, 1969b, 1969c), Gazzaniga (1967, 1970, 1972, 1978), and Sperry (1968a, 1968b, 1974, 1976, 1977a) provide a good entry to the empirical research and a fair sampling of the philosophical reflections of the experimenters. For a more extensive bibliography, see Bogen (1969c) for articles through 1968; for papers after 1968, consult the UCLA Brain Information Service bibliographies on split-brain studies. For an up-to-date record, the best recourse is a computerized search by MEDLARS II in the National Library of Medicine's National Interaction Retrieval Service.

The general point of view expressed in this paper is most like that of MacKay (1966a), though it is argued for in a completely different way. There are also points of contact between my views and those of Wilkes (1978), which I first saw after the penultimate version of the present paper was completed. Again, the views we share are largely based on different considerations.

2. Bogen (1969b), Gazzaniga (1967, 1970, 1972), Geschwind (1965b), Sperry (1966, 1968a, 1968b, 1974, 1977a).

3. A good deal of split-brain research concerns lateral specialization and cerebral dominance. Roughly, inferences are made from the performance of split-brain patients on various tasks to the presumed special abilities of each hemisphere and the dominance of one hemisphere over the other in controlling certain behavior in intact human beings. The present work is not concerned with these studies. For a straightforward presentation of some of the difficulties involved, see Kinsbourne (1974b), Liberman (1974), Broadbent (1974), and Whitaker and Ojemann (1977). The dichotomies listed in the text are a fairly mild sample. Left/right hemisphere differences have been associated with the distinction between female and male, Western and Eastern philosophy, Anglo and Chicano thought patterns; and the right hemisphere has been proclaimed the seat of the Freudian unconscious. See Bradshaw and Nettleton (1981).

4. Puccetti (1973a, 1973b, 1977a, 1977b).

5. Nagel (1971).

6. This is the operation Vogel and Bogen performed. In other operations undertaken for the same therapeutic purposes, the anterior commissure is spared (Wilson et al., 1977) or the corpus callosum is only partially sectioned (Gordon et al., 1971). The psychological results of these two types of operation differ from those of the operation performed by Vogel and Bogen.

7. Sperry (1974), p. 6.

8. Akelaitis (1941a, 1941b, 1941c, 1943, 1944).

9. The "optimistic" version, due to Lashley, was that the function of the corpus callosum was purely mechanical—to keep the hemispheres from sagging.

10. Sperry (1968a), p. 318.

11. However, the right hemisphere does receive some information about the right visual field; and the left about the left. Information picked up by so-called "ambient vision," e.g., the appearance of a light or dark stimulus, the location and orientation of a stimulus, and its direction and speed, is available to both hemispheres, presumably as a result of undivided subcortical mechanisms (Trevarthen and Sperry, 1973).

12. The major hemisphere is the one which controls speech, the minor the one which does not. In most people, the left hemisphere is the major hemisphere, the right the minor. In some left-handers, speech is controlled by the right hemisphere; and in a small number of people, speech is controlled by either hemisphere. I usually use 'right/left' where, in the interests of precision, I should use 'minor/major.'

13. Sperry (1968a), pp. 318–319; Sperry (1968b), pp. 730–733.

14. Sperry (1968a, 1968b, 1970), Gazzaniga (1967, 1970, 1972).

15. See Sperry et al. (1969) for a full description of the syndrome.

16. Gazzaniga et al. (1975); Gordon et al. (1971); Sperry (1974).

17. Sperry (1974).

18. No one thinks that people with either right or left hemispherectomies lack minds comfortably characterizable as human.

19. Sperry (1967), p. 717.

20. See Nagel (1971), p. 409; Puccetti (1973a), p. 351; and Puccetti (1977b), p. 131.

21. Sperry (1977a); Sperry et al. (1979).

22. "We know beyond a shadow of a doubt that it is this brain structure [the corpus callosum] which relates the psychological, conscious experiences of one hemisphere to the other." (Gazzaniga, 1972, p. 316.)

23. Eccles (1970).

24. MacKay (1966).

25. Bogen (1969b).

26. Although there is no good reason to doubt that some conscious mental activity is associated with the minor hemisphere, simple experiments like the "key ring" experiment leave open the possibility that there is no simultaneous conscious activity in each hemisphere. While the extent to which both hemispheres are simultaneously conscious may be overestimated (Kinsbourne, 1974b), that they sometimes are is established by the experiments done by Levy et al. (1972). I do not pursue this line because (1) temporal alternations in consciousness would pose as good an argument for two minds as simultaneity and (2) even if, as Eccles supposes, all minor hemisphere processes were unconscious, it is still possible to argue that split-brain patients have two minds. All that is required is that we be willing to ascribe propositional attitudes to the minor hemisphere and explain the behavior it controls in terms of them. The argument is sketched on pp. 38–39.

27. Nagel (1971), pp. 406–408.

28. It is important to notice that no questions are being begged. In the "key ring" experiment, there are two simultaneous conscious experiences associated with a particular human being, the split-brain patient. If they fail to meet the proposed necessary condition, I say that the split-brain patient lacks unity of consciousness or has a disunified consciousness. By itself, this is completely neutral on the question of whether the split-brain patient contains two separate conscious entities (minds, subjects of experience, or persons), each of which enjoys complete unity of consciousness. Of course, if the split-brain patient did contain two such entities, that would explain why he lacks unity of consciousness on the proposed necessary condition.

29. I have not seen any studies on the effects of commissurotomy on long-term memory in human beings. I suspect that this is because it is assumed that there are two independent short-term memories, like the supposed two independent spheres of consciousness; and so there must be two independent long-term memories as well, even though they have largely similar contents.

30. Grice (1941), p. 344.

31. See Gazzaniga (1967, 1970). "Cross-cuing" is the use by one hemisphere of sensory information derived from responses initiated by the other. One simple case of "cross-cuing" appeared in an early experiment, designed to test whether the right hemisphere could respond verbally to simple red or green stimuli. At first, when the stimuli were presented exclusively to the right hemisphere, the subject would guess the colors at a chance level. But after a few trials, the scores improved whenever a second guess was allowed. Gazzaniga's (1967, p. 27) explanation is the following: "We soon caught on to the strategy the patient used. If a red light was flashed and the patient by chance guessed

red, he would stick with that answer. If the flashed light was red, and the patient by chance guessed green, he would frown, shake his head, and then say, 'Oh no, I meant red.' What was happening was that the right hemisphere saw the red light and heard the left hemisphere make the guess 'green.' Knowing that the answer was wrong, the right hemisphere precipitated a frown and a shake of the head, which in turn cued in the left hemisphere to the fact that the answer was wrong and that it had better correct itself." The extent to which behavioral integration in split-brain patients and others without corpus callosums is a product of "cross-cuing," as opposed to other mechanisms for bilateral duplication of information, is a matter for debate. See Trevarthen and Sperry (1973); Trevarthen (1974a, 1974c); Ettlinger et al. (1972); Lehmann and Lampe (1970).

32. See footnote 36.

33. The same information may be more perspicuous in tabular form:

Subject	Situation	Neural Mechanisms	Behavior	Consciousness
1. Split-brain	Experimental, i.e., lateralized input and controls against cross-cuing and independent duplication	Extra-commissural, excluding cross-cuing and independent duplication	Non-integrated	Disunified
2. Normal	Experimental	Commissural	Integrated	Unified
3. Split-brain	Everyday	Extra-commissural	Integrated	?
4. Normal	Everyday	Commissural and extra-commissural	Integrated	Unified

34. From the start, the literature on split-brain patients has emphasized the normalcy of their everyday behavior after recovery from the operation. I will rely heavily on two facts: (1) that the behavioral integration of split-brain patients is roughly on a par with ours in ordinary circumstances and (2) that clear and compelling evidence for disunity of consciousness is obtained only in the relevant experimental situations. But my account does not require that there be no differences in behavioral integration between us and the split-brain patients outside the laboratory, nor does it require that split-brain patients exhibit disunity of consciousness only within. Bearing this in mind, a few qualifications and caveats are in order. Some split-brain patients do sometimes behave abnormally in everyday life, and some of this behavior may be the result of commissurotomy. Most of this abnormal behavior and the presumed underlying deficits, e.g., in short-term memory, have no bearing on unity of consciousness and mind; and they do not seriously affect overall behavioral integration. I have simply disregarded these abnormalities. In the early split-brain literature, there were some anecdotal reports of intermanual conflict. [See Lishman (1971), pp. 188–191, for a summary and discussion.] Although such reports have largely disappeared from the literature, some patients do continue to report intermanual conflicts, e.g., lack of control over the left hand and even being slapped awake by the left hand. (I am indebted to Puccetti for furnishing me with some reports which were obtained by Dimond.) These conflicts are failures of behavioral integration outside the relevant experimental situations, and they may bear upon the unity of consciousness and mind of the split-brain patient. If, for example, the two-minds account were independently established, it would be tempting to try to interpret them as acts of rebellion by the usually docile right hemisphere. But, by themselves, the conflicts are hardly compelling evidence for a division of consciousness and can be accounted for in a variety of ways which do not imply that they are the result of a disunified consciousness. Nor do they signal a significant breakdown in overall behavioral integration. It is also unknown whether the conflicts are the result of commissurotomy or brain damage caused by epilepsy.

35. The rhetorical question is backed by an intuition I have often heard expressed that unity or disunity of consciousness (or mind) *should not* be a function of purely en-

vironmental variables or relatively peripheral events like eye movement. For an evalua-
tion of the intuition, see footnote 42.

36. But it is not, Sperry has informed me (personal correspondence), what he intended. His own view is more complex and, for several reasons, difficult to make precise.
Along with his split-brain research, Sperry has developed a theory of consciousness
(1952, 1969, 1976). According to the theory, consciousness is an emergent property of
large-scale brain processes, which are themselves picked out by the functional role they
play in brain dynamics. These functional units both influence and are influenced by
more molecular neural activity. No isomorphism is presumed to exist between the properties of conscious experience and those of the underlying brain processes. It is this
"functional derivative " view of consciousness which lies behind the criterion stated. The
criterion itself—"A cerebral process acts as a conscious entity . . . because it functions
organizationally as a unit"—is vague and unsatisfactory. Unsatisfactory because, whatever the precise explanation of functioning organizationally as a unit, there are presumably many brain processes which so function without being conscious. So the criterion
is, at best, a necessary condition for a brain process being conscious. More importantly,
the notion of a functional unit, which comes from the theory of consciousness, is too
vague for present purposes. When the split-brain patient obtains dual neural representations of 'key ring' as the result of eye movement, have we one unit or two, one conscious
process or two? As I understand Sperry, the brain processes which constitute the functional units will be specified in terms of the psychological functions they perform. If
this is so, Sperry is certainly right in thinking that nothing in his theory of consciousness
excludes functional units comprised of causally unrelated brain processes. But then the
dual representations of 'key ring' may be a single functional unit, and on the criterion,
there may be a single conscious process of seeing 'key ring' (see pp. 23-24) and 40-43
above). On the other hand, if a brain process functions as a unit only if its components
are causally connected in a fairly direct way, the dual representations of 'key ring' will
not function as a unit, and there will be, on the criterion, two conscious experiences, not
one. Although nothing in Sperry's theory of consciousness requires such a restriction, it
is compatible with his firm rejection of any isomorphism between the properties of
conscious experience and the underlying brain processes. Without the restriction, I do
not see any well-motivated interpretation of 'functional unit' which ensures that split-
brain patients always have a divided consciousness. Thus my assumption of the restriction makes it harder, not easier, to argue that the consciousness of split-brain patients is
not always divided.

Another complicating factor is that Sperry often writes as though the mechanisms for
independent duplication actually unified consciousness, although his official position is
that the split-brain patient always has a dual consciousness with largely overlapping contents. "Our interpretation does not preclude a retention in the bisected brain of right-left
unity in some aspects and levels of conscious experience. This is ensured in part by bilateral sensory representation in each hemisphere as is the case, for example, with facial
sensibility" (1976, p. 172). This may just mean that such mechanisms assure similar conscious experiences in each hemisphere, as is suggested by his next sentence: "We pre-
sume, however, by extrapolation, that these unified 'whole face' experiences in each
hemisphere are cut off from their counterparts in the opposite hemisphere" (1976,
p. 172). But Sperry often makes similar remarks without qualification. If the mechanisms for independent duplication do produce single conscious experiences, the "two
minds" interpretation of split-brain patients is in trouble because (1) there will be little
reason to claim that the consciousness of split-brain patients is always disunified and (2)
two minds will not be enough (see p. 24 above).

37. This echoes von Hartmann (1931, pp. 117-118): "We may lay down . . . as a
principle: Separate material parts give separate consciousness . . . if the brains of two
men could be effectively joined by a bridge of nervous matter, as the two halves of the
human brain are joined by the corpus callosum, the two men would have a single, common consciousness."

38. The behavioral integration of split-brain patients is itself evidence for the redundancy. See also LeDoux et al. (1977) and Kinsbourne (1974a).

39. This hypothesis is intended only to make a conceptual point about Sperry's

criterion. But it is as tame as some possibilities more seriously considered (see, for example, Zangwill, 1974, p. 268), and it would explain why the everyday behavior of split-brain patients is as integrated as it is so quickly after the operation.

40. There is a tendency to think that such theoretical considerations are inappropriate or, at best, appropriate only because we cannot get inside the split-brain patient's psyche. He must know whether his consciousness is unified; and if I were to have a commissurotomy, I would know too. Thus, in 1911, long before commissurotomies were done, the British psychologist William McDougall tried to strike a bargain with Sherrington that, if he became the victim of an incurable disease, Sherrington should cut through his corpus callosum. "If the physiologists are right, the result should be a split personality. If I am right, my consciousness will remain a unitary consciousness" (Zangwill, 1974, p. 265). It would not help to have a commissurotomy. It is possible, I suppose, that the patient could learn that his consciousness is disunified under experimental conditions, although this does not, in fact, happen. But the evidence on which the patient must rely is the same as that available to the experimenter; and his decision on whether he has a disunified consciousness would depend upon the same behavioral and theoretical conditions. Disunity in consciousness is obviously not, nor could it be, a fact introspectively disclosed.

41. See pp. 43–45.

42. As far as I can see, the only motivation is the feeling that environmental and relatively peripheral events should not divide/unify consciousness (or even multiply minds) in the way it appears they might if the causal principle were abandoned. Nagel (1971, p. 408) comes close to expressing this view, though about minds rather than consciousness: "There is nothing about the experimental situation that might be expected to produce a fundamental internal change in the patient. In fact it produces no anatomical changes and merely elicits a noteworthy set of symptoms. So unusual an event as a· mind's popping in and out of existence would have to be explained by something more than its explanatory convenience." I tend to agree about minds, but there is nothing implausible in thinking that environmental events, like tachistoscopic presentation, may disunify consciousness. Unity, even our unity, depends upon certain mechanisms; and mechanisms can fail under some environmental conditions and not under others. On the view being considered, the mechanisms available for unifying the consciousness of split-brain patients fail in the experimental situations where independent duplication is controlled against. But that hardly means they do not work at all.

43. Fodor (1975).

44. Grice (1975).

45. See pp. 33–35.

46. Trevarthen and Sperry (1973).

47. Recently Sperry has shown some ambivalence about the concepts of mind and person, claiming that they need to be either redefined or more precisely defined. "Already it makes little sense, employing past definitions, to argue about how many 'minds' or 'persons' are present in the bisected brain" (Sperry, 1976, p. 172). But this is tempered a great deal by his later remark that "regardless of terminology, however, the question of whether the normal intact brain contains only one unified realm of conscious awareness or alternatively maintains separate conscious systems, or minds, one centered in each hemisphere, poses a rather clear dichotomy that should be subject eventually to a definite empirical answer" (Sperry, 1977a, p. 116).

48. Thus, in the example in footnote 31, the right hemisphere would be taken to frown and shake the head in order to inform the left that its answer was incorrect and the left hemisphere to await a signal from its silent partner.

49. See, for example, Sperry (1977a), p. 105.

50. Zaidel (1975); Sperry (1977a); Sperry et al. (1979).

51. Saul and Sperry (1968); Sperry (1974); Ettlinger et al. (1972, 1974); Lehmann and Lampe (1970).

52. Sperry (1974), p. 10.

53. LeDoux et al. (1977). In fact, the general postoperative improvement of the patient and lack of any deficits lead the authors to conclude that "these results demonstrate

that the processing of complex information is not necessarily dependent upon the integrity of the corpus callosum, but rather suggest that cognitive functioning is largely an intrahemispheric process" (p. 102).

54. Sperry (1974), p. 10.

55. This would be highly implausible if one assumes a basically Cartesian account of mind: that all mental events are conscious and a single mind is introspectively aware of all its simultaneous contents. But one's view of mind can be influenced by the fact that psychological processes and events, most of which are unconscious, serve, *inter alia*, to explain behavior. It *may* turn out that unity of consciousness is an epiphenomenon. For example, if one thought that interhemispheric integrity is necessary for unity of consciousness, the findings of LeDoux et al. (1977) suggest that unity of consciousness is irrelevant to cognitive function. And, if unity of consciousness is an epiphenomenon, it seems possible to maintain that a single mind may have a totally disunified consciousness with largely overlapping contents. See pp. 33–43 for a more extensive discussion.

56. Puccetti (1973a).

57. Puccetti (1973a), p. 351; Puccetti (1977b), p. 131.

58. See pp. 43–45.

59. There are straightforward empirical problems as well about the inference from hemispheric performance in commissurotomy patients to hemispheric function in a normal intact brain. Since commissurotomy is a last resort for intractable epilepsy, split-brain patients have probably suffered some, perhaps extensive, brain damage before the operation. Moreover the amount of hemispheric activity in the intact brain is inhibited by activity in the other hemispheres. See Kinsbourne (1974b), Broadbent (1974), and Whitaker and Ojemann (1977).

60. A possible exception to the claim in the text, due to Gazzaniga (1972) and cited by Puccetti (1975), is that some, but not all, brain-damaged nonaphasic subjects exhibited the following behavior: While their left hemispheres were anesthetized, an object was placed in their hands. After the anesthesia wore off, the subjects verbally denied knowing what was in their left hand, although they were able to point left-handed to the correct object. One problem is whether the behavior exhibited implicates conscious mental processes. The behavior of Gazzaniga's subjects seems to be no more compelling evidence for conscious mental processes than the analogous behavior of the subject in Weiskrantz et al. (1974). In the case of "blindsight," are we to suppose that there is conscious visual and memory experience underlying the subject's remarkable performance? I do not, of course, deny that there is overwhelming evidence for the existence of unconscious mental processes whose products influence our behavior and sometimes conflict with our conscious beliefs and desires. Nor do I deny that a normal commissure-intact person may, under some possible conditions, have a disunified consciousness (see pp. 30–32 and 35–43 above).

Puccetti (1977a, p. 454; 1977b, p. 136) does propose a relatively direct test for duality of consciousness in normals. The test involves questioning a subject, whose left hemisphere is anesthetized, about the simultaneity of some flashing lights observed before anesthetization. Although he had previously judged them to be simultaneous, the dual-consciousness hypothesis predicts that he may deny that they were because the neural representations of the lights in the right hemisphere were not simultaneous. Temporarily freed from the domination of the left, the right hemisphere may report the true temporal order of its experiences. Perhaps this would be the outcome of the experiment, in which case we would have some behavioral evidence favoring dual consciousness in normals; but possible outcomes are not outcomes. There are, of course, a number of right hemispheres permanently freed from the left. So far as I know, the hemispherectomy cases have not produced any memory reports favoring dual consciousness. Puccetti has informed me that he has abandoned the test because new data indicate that the left hemisphere would report what the right hemisphere sees, and so no discrepancy rectomy cases have not produced any memory reports favoring dual consciousness.

61. At least to me. Puccetti (1977a, p. 453; 1977b, p. 135) argues, in effect, that if we had a unified consciousness, we ought to have duplicate visual fields, side by side, because there is neurological representation of the entire visual field in each hemisphere. And, since we do not, we must be compounds of two conscious entities. He does not, however, explain why dual neural representation should lead to double vision.

Since the first printing, Puccetti (1981) has presented further agreements for mental duality. See the Open Peer Commentary on his article and the author's response.

62. Nagel (1971).

63. Nagel (1971), p. 407.

64. Nagel (1971), p. 410.

65. Wada and Rasmussen (1960); Blume et al. (1973); Serafetinedes et al. (1965).

66. Perhaps a more Cartesian account would. It is surprising how Cartesian Sperry is, tending throughout his writings to identify minds and selves with realms of conscious awareness. See, for example, Sperry (1976), p. 166, for an identification of mental properties with conscious properties.

67. Nagel (1974).

68. See footnote 40.

69. Perry (1976).

70. Perry (1976), p. 70.

71. So I agree with Nagel (1971, p. 410) that "our own unity may be nothing absolute, but merely another case of integration, more or less effective, in the control system of a complex organism."

72. Sutcliffe and Jones (1962), p. 260. The case was extensively described by Dr. Weir Mitchell, whose report is quoted in James (1950), Volume 1, pp. 381-384. My in- a single structure of propositional attitudes. As reported the actual case is relatively clean, but a few details would have to be "fictionalized" in order to have an unblemished illustration.

73. But not so dramatically as one might expect. The focusing of the subject's eyes on the fixation point, his positioning himself relative to the testing apparatus, and so on are explicable in the normal way.

74. This is what the explanation requires. The mere belief that he did not see 'key' or 'ring' is not enough for several reasons. One is that, if 'x believes that not-p' is allowed to substitute for 'it is false that x believes that p,' the explanatory schema will predict incompatible actions when the agent has contradictory beliefs. Another is that the pattern of explanation warrants an indefinitely large number of counterfactuals of the form 'If he were asked . . . , he would not point to/say . . . .' So, for example, he would not point to 'jacaranda.' And it is not true that he believes he did not see 'jacaranda,' although it is true that he does not believe he saw 'jacaranda.'

75. This failure is about all that split-brain patients have in common with some other cases, sometimes offered as comparisons, in which people apparently hold contradictory beliefs, e.g., akrasia. The explanation for the conflicting beliefs in these cases and those of the split-brain patients, and so for the failure of the usual explanations of behavior, is entirely different. However puzzling it may be, it is a fact of life that human beings sometimes believe or desire that p and also not-p. It is also a fact that the description of the *content* of one's visual experience, Puccetti (1973a) to the contrary, sometimes requires a self-contradictory phrase—as, for example, the description of one's visual experience when viewing a Penrose triangle or a staircase designed by Escher.

76. Trevarthen (1974c), Sperry (1974).

77. Fodor (1975), pp. 9-26.

78. This is the extent of my agreement with Sperry that there will be a definite empirical answer to the question of whether we have two minds, as there presumably already is to the question of whether split-brain patients have two minds. See Sperry (1977a), p. 116.

79. Plato (1945), pp. 129-138 (434d-441c).

BIBLIOGRAPHY

Akelaitis, A. J. (1941a) Psychobiological studies following section of the corpus callosum: a preliminary report, *American Journal of Psychiatry* 97, pp. 1147-1157.

Akelaitis, A. J. (1941b) Studies on the corpus callosum. VIII. The effects of partial and complete section of the corpus callosum on psychopathic epileptics, *American Journal of Psychiatry* 98, pp. 409-414.

Akelaitis, A. J. (1941c) Studies on the corpus callosum. II. The higher visual functions in each homonymous field following complete section of the corpus callosum, *Archives of Neurological Psychiatry* 45, pp. 788-796.

Akelaitis, A. J. (1943) Studies on the corpus callosum. VII. Study of language functions (tactile and visual lexia and graphia) unilaterally following section of the corpus callosum, *Journal of Neuropathology and Experimental Neurology* 2, pp. 226-262.

Akelaitis, A. J. (1944) Study on gnosis, praxia, and language following section of corpus callosum and anterior commissure, *Journal of Neurosurgery* 1, pp. 94-102.

Amaded, M., R. A. Roemer, and C. Shagass: (1977) Can callosal speed of transmission be inferred from verbal reaction times? *Biological Psychiatry* 12, pp. 289-297.

Anderson, S. L. (1976) Consciousness and numerical identity of the person, *Philosophical Studies* 30, pp. 1-10.

Austin, G., W. Hayward, and S. Rouke (1974) A note on the problem of conscious man and cerebral disconnection by hemispherectomy, in M. Kinsbourne and W. L. Smith (eds.), *Hemispheric Disconnection and Cerebral Function*, Thomas, Springfield, pp. 95-114.

Bennett, J. (1967) The simplicity of the soul, *Journal of Philosophy* 54, pp. 648-660.

Bennett, J. (1974) Mental disunity, in J. Bennett, *Kant's Dialectic*, Cambridge University Press, Cambridge, pp. 87-90.

Berlucchi, G. (1974) Cerebral dominance and interhemispheric communication in normal man, in F. O. Schmitt and F. G. Worden (eds.), *The Neurosciences*, Third Study Program, M.I.T. Press, Cambridge, pp. 65-69.

Blume, W. T., J. D. Grabow, F. L. Darley, and A. E. Aronson (1973) Intracarotid test of language and memory before temporal lobectomy for seizure control, *Neurology* 23, pp. 812-819.

Bogen, J. E. (1969a) The other side of the brain. I. Dysgraphia and dyscopia following cerebral commissurotomy, *Bulletin of the Los Angeles Neurological Society* 34, pp. 73-105.

Bogen, J. E. (1969b) The other side of the brain. II. An appositional mind, *Bulletin of the Los Angeles Neurological Society* 34, pp. 135-162.

Bogen, J. E., and G. M. Bogen (1969c) The other side of the brain. III. The corpus callosum and creativity, *Bulletin of the Los Angeles Neurological Society* 34, pp. 191-220.

Bogen, J. E. (1977) Further discussion of split-brains and hemispheric capabilities, *British Journal for the Philosophy of Science* 28, pp. 281-286.

Bradshaw, J. L., and Nettleton, N. C. (1981) The nature of hemispheric specialization in man, *The Behavioral and Brain Sciences* 4, pp. 51-91.

Broadbent, D. E. (1974) Division of function and integration of behavior, in F. O. Schmitt and F. G. Worden (eds.), *The Neurosciences*, Third Study Program, M.I.T. Press, Cambridge, pp. 31-41.

Burklund, C. W., and Smith, A. (1977) Language and the cerebral hemispheres, *Neurology* 27, pp. 627-633.

Critchley, M. (1972) Interhemispheric partnership and interhemispheric rivalry, in M. Critchley, J. L. O'Leary, and B. Jennett (eds.), *Scientific Foundations of Neurology*, Heinemann, London, pp. 216-221.

Dennett, D. C. (1969) *Content and Consciousness*, Routledge and Kegan Paul, London.

de Sousa, R. (1976) Rational homunculi, in A. I. Rorty (ed.), *The Identities of Persons*, University of California Press, Berkeley, pp. 217-238.

Dewitt, L. (1975) Consciousness, mind, self: the implications of the split-brain studies, *British Journal for the Philosophy of Science* 27, pp. 41-47.

Dimond, S. J. (1975) The disconnection syndromes, *Modern Trends in Neurology* 6, pp. 35-57.

Dimond, S. J. (1976a) Brain circuits for consciousness, *Brain, Behavior, and Evolution* 13, pp. 376-395.

Dimond, S. J. (1976b) Depletion of attentional capacity after total commissurotomy in man, *Brain* 99, pp. 347-356.

Eccles, J. (1970) The brain and the unity of conscious experience, in J. Eccles, *Facing Reality: Philosophical Adventures by a Brain Scientist*, Springer-Verlag, New York, pp. 63-84.

Ettlinger, G., C. B. Blakemore, A. D. Milner, and J. Wilson (1972) Agenesis of the corpus callosum: a behavioral investigation, *Brain* 95, pp. 327-346.

Ettlinger, G., C. B. Blakemore, A. D. Milner, and J. Wilson (1974) Agenesis of the corpus callosum: a further behavioral investigation, *Brain* 97, pp. 225-234.

Fodor, J. A. (1975) *The Language of Thought*, Crowell, New York.

Galin, D., and R. E. Ornstein: (1975) Hemispheric specialization and the duality of consciousness, in H. J. Widroe (ed.), *Human Behavior and Brain Function*, Thomas, Springfield, pp. 3-23.

Gazzaniga, M. S. (1967) The split brain in man, *Scientific American* 217, pp. 24-29.

Gazzaniga, M. S. (1970) *The Bisected Brain*, Appleton-Century-Crofts, New York.

Gazzaniga, M. S. (1972) One brain—two minds, *American Scientist* 60, pp. 311-317.

Gazzaniga, M. S. (1978) On dividing the self: speculations from brain research, in W. den Hartog Jager, G. Bruyn, and A. Heijstee (eds.), *Neurology, Proceedings of the 11th World Congress of Neurology,* International Congress Series No. 434, Amsterdam, pp. 233-244.

Gazzaniga, M. S., and J. E. LeDoux (1978) *The Integrated Mind*, Plenum, New York.

Gazzaniga, M. S., G. L. Risse, S. P. Springer, E. Clark, and D. H. Wilson (1975) Psychologic and neurologic consequences of partial and complete cerebral commissurotomy, *Neurology* 25, pp. 10-15.

Gazzaniga, **M. S.**, Le Doux, J. E., and Wilson, D. H. (1977) Language, praxis, and the right hemisphere: clue to some mechanisms of consciousness,*Neurology*, 27, pp. 1144-1147.

Gazzaniga, M. S., Volpe, B. T., Smylie, C. S., Wilson, D. H., and Le Doux, J. E. (1979) Plasticity in speech organization following commissurotomy, *Brain* 102, pp. 805-815.

Geschwind, N. (1965a) Disconnexion syndromes in animals and man. Part I, *Brain* 88, pp. 237-294.

Geschwind, N. (1965b) Disconnexion syndromes in animals and man. Part II, *Brain* 88, pp. 585-644.

Gordon, H. W. (1974) Olfaction and cerebral separation, in M. Kinsbourne and W. L. Smith (eds.), *Hemispheric Disconnection and Cerebral Function*, Thomas, Springfield, pp. 137-154.

Gordon, H. W., J. E. Bogen, and R. W. Sperry (1971) Absence of deconnexion syndrome in two patients with partial section of the neocommissures, *Brain* 94, pp. 327-336.

Gordon, W. H., and R. W. Sperry (1969) Lateralization of olfactory perception in the surgically separated hemispheres of man, *Neuropsychologia* 7, pp. 111-120.

Greenwood, P., D. H. Wilson, and M. S. Gazzaniga: (1977) Dream report following commissurotomy, *Cortex* 13, pp. 311-316.

Grice, H. P. (1941) Personal identity, *Mind* 50, pp. 330-350.

Grice, H. P. (1975) Method in philosophical psychology (from the banal to the bizarre), *Proceedings and Addresses of the American Philosophical Association* 48, pp. 23-53.

Hoppe, K. D. (1977) Split brains and psychoanalysis, *Psychoanalytic Quarterly* 46, pp. 220-244.

Hurwitz, L. J. (1971) Evidence for restitution of function and development of new function in cases of brain bi-section, *Cortex* 7, pp. 401-409.

James, W. (1950) *The Principles of Psychology,* Volumes 1 and 2, Dover, New York.

Jeeves, M. A. (1972) Further psychological studies of the effects of agenesis of the corpus callosum in man and neonatal sectioning of the corpus callosum in animals, in J. Cernacek and F. Podivinsky (eds.), *Cerebral Interhemispheric Relations*, Vydatelstvo Slovenskej Akademie Vied, Bratislava, pp. 253-265.

Joynt, R. J. (1974) The corpus callosum: history of thought regarding its function, in M. Kinsbourne and W. L. Smith (eds.), *Hemispheric Disconnection and Cerebral Function*, Thomas, Springfield, pp. 117-125.

Joynt, R. J. (1977) Inattention syndromes in split-brain man, *Advances in Neurology* 18, pp. 33-39.

Kinsbourne, M. (1974a) Lateral interactions in the brain, in M. Kinsbourne and W. L. Smith (eds.), *Hemispheric Disconnection and Cerebral Function*, Thomas, Springfield,, pp. 239-259.

Kinsbourne, M. (1974b) Mechanisms of hemisphere interaction in man, in M. Kinsbourne and M. L. Smith (eds.), *Hemispheric Disconnection and Cerebral Function*, Thomas, Springfield, pp. 260-285.

Kinsbourne, M. (1974c) Cerebral control and mental evolution, in M. Kinsbourne and M. L. Smith (eds.), *Hemispheric Disconnection and Cerebral Function* Thomas, Springfield, pp. 286-289.

Kreuter, C., M. Kinsbourne, and C. Trevarthen (1972) Are deconnected cerebral hemispheres independent channels? *Neuropsychologia* 10, pp. 453-461.

Kumar, S. (1977) Short term memory for a nonverbal tactual task after cerebral commissurotomy, *Cortex* 13, pp. 55-61.

LeDoux, J. E., G. L. Risse, S. P. Spring, D. H. Wilson, and M. S. Gazzaniga (1977) Cognition and commissurotomy, *Brain* 100, pp. 87-104.

Lehmann, H. J., and H. Lampe (1970) Observations on the interhemispheric transmission of information in 9 patients with corpus callosum defect, *European Neurology* 4, pp. 129-147.

Levy, J. (1972) Lateral specialization of the human brain: behavioral manifestations and possible evolutionary basis, in J. A. Kiger (ed.), *The Biology of Behavior*, Oregon State University Press, Corvallis, pp. 159-180.

Levy, J. (1974a) Cerebral asymmetries as manifested in split-brain man, in M. Kinsbourne and M. L. Smith (eds.), *Hemispheric Disconnection and Cerebral Function*, Thomas, Springfield, pp. 165-183.

Levy, J. (1974b) Psychobiological implications of bilateral asymmetry, in S. J. Dimond and J. G. Beaumont (eds.), *Hemisphere Function in the Human Brain*, Wiley, New York, pp. 121-183.

Levy, J. (1977) Manifestations and implications of shifting hemi-inattention in commissurotomy patients, *Advances in Neurology* 18, pp. 83-92.

Levy, J., and C. Trevarthen (1976) Metacontrol of Hemispheric function in human split-brain patients, *Journal of Experimental Psychology: Human Perception and Performance* 2, pp. 299-312.

Levy, J., C. Trevarthen, and R. W. Sperry (1972) Perception of bilateral chimeric figures following hemisphere deconnection, *Brain* 95, pp. 61-78.

Liberman, A. M. (1974) The specialization of the language hemisphere, in F. O. Schmitt and F. G. Worden (eds.), *The Neurosciences,* Third Study Program, M.I.T. Press, Cambridge, pp. 43-56.

Lishman, W. A. (1971) Emotion, consciousness, and will after brain bisection in man, *Cortex* 7, pp. 181-192.

MacKay, D. M. (1966a) Discussion, in J. C. Eccles (ed.), *Brain and Conscious Experience*, Springer-Verlag, Heidelberg, pp. 312-313.

MacKay, D. M. (1966b) Cerebral organization and the conscious control of action, in J. C. Eccles (ed.), *Brain and Conscious Experience*, Springer-Verlag, Heidelberg, pp. 422-444.

MacKenzie, N. (1977) Heaps, bits, hunks, and minds, unpublished.

Milner, B. (1974) Hemispheric specialization: scope and limits, in F. O. Schmitt and F. G. Worden (eds.), *The Neurosciences*, Third Study Program, M.I.T. Press, Cambridge, pp. 75-89.

Milner, B., L. Taylor, and R. W. Sperry (1968) Lateralized suppression of dichotically presented digits after commissural section in man, *Science* 161, pp. 184-186.

Nagel, T. (1971) Brain bisection and the unity of consciousness, *Synthese* 22, pp. 396-413.

Nagel, T. (1974) What is it like to be a bat?, *Philosophical Review* 83, pp. 435-450.

Nebes, R. (1974) Hemispheric specialization in commissurotomized man, *Psychological Bulletin* 81, pp. 1-14.

Perry, J. (1972) Can the self divide? *Journal of Philosophy* 69, pp. 463-488.

Perry, J. (ed.) (1975) *Personal Identity*, University of California Press, Berkeley.

Perry, J. (1976) The importance of being identical, in A. O. Rorty (ed.), *The Identities of Persons*, University of California Press, Berkeley, pp. 67-90.

Plato (1945) *The Republic*, translated with introduction and notes by F. M. Cornford, Oxford University Press, New York.

Puccetti, R. (1973a) Brain bisection and personal identity, *British Journal for the Philosophy of Science* 24, pp. 339–355.

Puccetti, R. (1973b) Multiple identity, *The Personalist* 54, pp. 203–215.

Puccetti, R. (1975) A reply to Professor Margolis, *Philosophy of Science* 42, pp. 281–285.

Puccetti, R.. (1976) The mute self: a reaction to Dewitt's alternative account of the split-brain data, *British Journal for the Philosophy of Science* 27, pp. 65–73.

Puccetti, R. (1977a) Bilerateral organization of consciousness in man, *Annals of the New York Academy of Sciences* 299, pp. 448–457.

Puccetti, R. (1977b) Sperry on consciousness: a critical appreciation, *The Journal of Medicine and Philosophy* 2, pp. 139–144.

Puccetti, R. (1981) The case for mental duality: evidence from split-brain data and other considerations, *The Behavioral and Brain Sciences* 4, pp. 93–123.

Rey, G. (1976) Survival, in A. O. Rorty (ed.), *The Identities of Persons*, University of California Press, Berkeley, pp. 41–66.

Risse, G. L., and Gazzaniga, M. S. 1978) Well-kept secrets of the right hemisphere: a carotid amytal study of restricted memory transfer, *Neurology* 28, pp. 950–953.

Robinson, D. N. (1976) What sort of persons are hemispheres? Another look at split-brain man, *British Journal for the Philosophy of Science* 27, pp. 73–78.

Saul, R., and R. W. Sperry (1968) Absence of commissurotomy symptoms with agenesis of the corpus callosum, *Neurology* 18, p. 307.

Serafetinedes, E. A., R. D. Hoare, and M. V. Driver (1965) Intracarotid sodium amylobarbitone and cerebral dominance for speech and consciousness, *Brain* 88, pp. 107–130.

Shaffer, J. (1977) Personal identity: the implications of brain bisection and brain transplants, *The Journal of Medicine and Philosophy* 2, pp. 147–161.

Sperry, R. W. (1952) Neurology and the mind-brain problem, *American Scientist* 40, pp. 291–312.

Sperry, R. W. (1966) Brain bisection and mechanisms of consciousness, in J. C. Eccles (ed.), *Brain and Conscious Experience*, Springer-Verlag, Heidelberg, pp. 298–313.

Sperry, R. W. (1967) Split-brain approach to learning problems, in G. C. Quarter, T. Melnechuk, and F. O. Schmitt (eds.), *The Neurosciences, a Study Program*, Rockefeller University Press, New York, pp. 714–722.

Sperry, R. W. (1968a) Mental unity following surgical disconnection of the cerebral hemispheres, *Harvey Lectures* 62, pp. 293–323.

Sperry, R. W. (1968b) Hemisphere deconnection and unity in conscious awareness, *American Psychologist* 23, pp. 723–733.

Sperry, R. W. (1969) A modified concept of consciousness, *Psychological Review* 76, pp. 532–536.

Sperry, R. W. (1970) Perception in the absence of the neocortical commissures, *Perception and Its Disorders* (Research Publication Association for Research in Nervous and Mental Disease) 48, pp. 123–138.

Sperry, R. W. (1974) Lateral specialization in the surgically separated hemispheres, in F. O. Schmitt and F. G. Worden (eds.), *The Neurosciences*, Third Study Program, M.I.T. Press, Cambridge, pp. 5–19.

Sperry, R. W. (1976) Mental phenomena as causal determinants in brain function, in G. C. Globus, G. Maxwell, and I. Savodnik (eds.), *Consciousness and the Brain: a Scientific and Philosophical Inquiry*, Plenum Press, New York, pp. 163–177.

Sperry, R. W. (1977a) Forebrain commissurotomy and conscious awareness, *The Journal of Medicine and Philosophy* 2, pp. 101–126.

Sperry, R. W. (1977b) Reply to Professor Puccetti, *The Journal of Medicine and Philosophy* 2, pp. 145–146.

Sperry, R. W., M. S. Gazzaniga, and J. E. Bogen (1969) Interhemispheric relationships: the neocortical commissures; syndromes of disconnection, in P. J. Vinken and G. W. Bruyn (eds.), *Handbook of Clinical Neurology*, Volume 4, North-Holland, New York, pp. 273–290.

Sperry, R. W., Zaidel, E., Zaidel, D. (1979) Self recognition and social awareness in the deconnected minor hemisphere, *Neuropsychologia* 17, pp. 153–166.

Sutcliffe, J. P., and J. Jones (1962) Personal identity, multiple personality, and hypnosis, *The International Journal of Clinical and Experimental Hypnosis* 10, pp. 231–269.

Trevarthen, C. (1970) Experimental evidence for a brain-stem contribution to visual perception in man, *Brain, Behavior, and Evolution* 3, pp. 338–352.

Trevarthen, C. (1972) Brain bisymmetry and the role of the corpus callosum in behavior and conscious experience, in J. Cernacek and F. Podivinsky (eds.), *Cerebral Interhemispheric Relations*, Vydatelstvo Slovenskej Akademie Vied, Bratislava, pp. 319–333.

Trevarthen, C. (1974a) Functional relations of disconnected hemispheres with the brain stem, and with each other: monkey and man, in M. Kinsbourne and W. L. Smith (eds.), *Hemispheric Disconnection and Cerebral Function*, Thomas, Springfield, pp. 187–207.

Trevarthen, C. (1974b) Cerebral embryology and the split-brain, in M. Kinsbourne and W. L. Smith (eds.), *Hemispheric Disconnection and Cerebral Function*, Thomas, Springfield, pp. 208–236.

Trevarthen, C. (1974c) Analysis of cerebral activities that generate and regulate consciousness in commissurotomy patients, in S. J. Dimond and J. G. Beaumont (eds.), *Hemisphere Function in the Human Brain*, Wiley, New York, pp. 235–263.

Trevarthen, C., and R. W. Sperry (1973) Perceptual unity of the ambient visual field in human commissurotomy patients, *Brain* 96, pp. 547–570.

von Hartmann, E. (1931) *Philosophy of the Unconscious*, Kegan Paul, Trench and Trubner, London.

Wada, J., and T. Rasmussen (1960) Intracarotid injection of sodium amytal for lateralization of cerebral speech dominance, *Journal of Neurosurgery* 17, pp. 266–282.

Weiskrantz, L., E. K. Warrington, M. D. Sanders, and J. Marshall (1974) Visual capacity in the hemianopic field following a restricted occipital ablation, *Brain* 97, pp. 709–728.

Whitaker, H. A., and G. A. Ojemann (1977) Lateralization of higher cortical functions: a critique, *Annals of the New York Academy of Sciences* 299, pp. 459–473.

Wilkes, K. V. (1978) Consciousness and commissurotomy, *Philosophy* 53, pp. 184–199.

Wilson, D. H., A. Reeves, M. S. Gazzaniga, and C. Culver (1977) Cerebral commissurotomy for control of intractable seizures, *Neurology* (Minneapolis) 27, pp. 708–715.

Zaidel, E. (1975) A technique for presenting lateralized visual input with prolonged exposure, *Vision Research* 15, pp. 283–289.

Zaidel, E. (1976) Auditory vocabulary of the right hemisphere following brain bisection or hemidecortication, *Cortex* 12, pp. 191–211.

Zangwill, O. L. (1974) Consciousness and the cerebral hemispheres, in S. J. Dimond and J. G. Beaumont (eds.), *Hemisphere Function in the Human Brain*, Wiley, New York, pp. 264–278.